AF333012

ENDOCRINOLOGY RESEARCH AND CLINICAL DEVELOPMENTS

ESTROGENS

BIOCHEMISTRY, THERAPEUTIC USES AND PHYSIOLOGICAL EFFECTS

ENDOCRINOLOGY RESEARCH AND CLINICAL DEVELOPMENTS

Additional books in this series can be found on Nova's website
under the Series tab.

Additional e-books in this series can be found on Nova's website
under the e-book tab.

ENDOCRINOLOGY RESEARCH AND CLINICAL DEVELOPMENTS

ESTROGENS

BIOCHEMISTRY, THERAPEUTIC USES AND PHYSIOLOGICAL EFFECTS

VITO J. THOMPSON

AND

ADRION E. WATSON

EDITORS

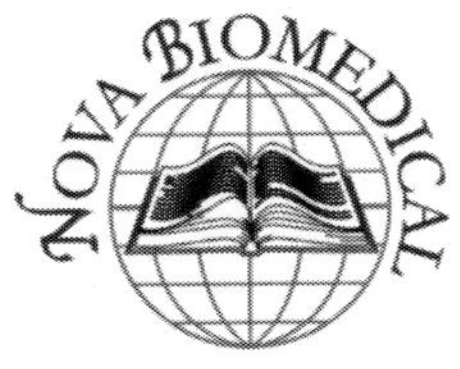

Nova Science Publishers, Inc.

New York

NOTICE TO THE READER

Library of Congress Cataloging-in-Publication Data

Library of Congress Control Number: 2012936710

ISBN: 978-1-62081-747-6

Published by Nova Science Publishers, Inc. † New York

CONTENTS

PREFACE

Estrogens are a family of hormones that potently regulate reproductive, cardiovascular, bone, brain, and other physiology by altering gene expression. In this book, the authors present topical research in the study of the biochemistry, therapeutic uses and physiological effects of hormones. Topics include the physiological effects of estrogen in fish and its application; estrogens in osteoarthritis and inflammation; estrogens as mediators of obesity-induced inflammation; the transcriptional effect of estrogens on gene expression; and the role of estrogens in regulating the gender disparity of hepatocellular carcinoma.

Chapter 1 - Obesity-related inflammation is a subject of great interest, not only for the exponential growth of obesity incidence but because obesity-driven inflammation may be an important instigator of the metabolic abnormalities that accompany the obese state. Estrogens have a role in metabolic control, through direct and indirect effects on the adipose tissue. The role of estrogens in inflammation and immune processes is now beginning to be unraveled with especial focus on cardiovascular and neurodegenerative disorders. In the case of the adipose tissue, effects of estrogens have remained rather unexploited regarding their possible association with the obese-related low-grade systemic inflammatory status. The adipose tissue is a source of estrogens and almost every cell type that composes it, including recruited inflammatory cells, may be a target for these hormones. In this regard, inflamematory cell recruitment into the adipose tissue in obese states has been considered central to the development the chronic inflammation associated with obesity. It has been suggested that subsets of infiltrating T cells may be a primary event in the initiation of adipose tissue inflammation. The recruitment of inflammatory cells to the site of inflammation is tightly governed by the expression of certain chemokines (e.g. MCP-1, MIP, RANTES) that play a central role in orchestrating the immune response. Therefore, interference with chemokine expression by estrogens can substantially alter the quality of the immune response and its outcomes. On the other hand, the tissue environment may change the differentiation path engaged by recruited cells into different activation sates, often with almost opposing consequences. For example, macrophages may be classically (M1) or alternatively (M2) activated, expressing a pro- and anti-inflammatory cytokine profile, respectively. Also T lymphocytes display the same alternative activation. T_H1 cells secrete the cytokines IL-2, IL-12, interferon-gamma and TNFalpha, whereas T_H2 cells secrete the cytokines IL-4, IL-5, IL-10 and IL-13. The interference on this differentiation path by estrogens may therefore substantially alter the inflame-matory response in the adipose tissue. Given the interplay of immune/ inflammatory and metabolic processes in the adipose tissue, estrogens may interfere with the tissue's endocrine function, which can be reflected on plasmatic efferent messages and affect distant targets. Moreover, estrogens may change tissue composition in inflammatory cells for the upper-mentioned modulation of leukocyte recruitment and differentiation. In this line, it has been proposed that knowing the source of adipose tissue derived inflammation and inflammatory cell infiltration or understanding how these processes can be modulated may help develop therapeutic tools to hamper the metabolic dysfunction associated with obesity. Here, we propose the role that estrogens play in obesity related inflammation through effects on adipose tissue and circulatory inflammatory cell number, type and functional properties. We will start to briefly overview estrogen metabolism, handling and signaling in the adipose tissue and we will present evidence of estrogen modulation of the immune system that may reflect on, or that occur directly within the adipose tissue. Furthermore, we will highlight the interference of adipose tissue estrogen signaling by xenobiotics with estrogen modulating-properties and their potential to modulate immune/inflammatory processes based on the adipose tissue and possibly promote adipose tissue dysfunction.

Chapter 2 - Behavioral studies that have evaluated the effects of meno-pause on some aspects of cognition suggest that certain impairments in cognitive performance are symptomatic of menopause. Cognitive deficits such as poor memory, inability to concentrate, deficits in abstract reasoning, attention and set-shifting flexibility, visuospatial ability, episodic memory and verbal fluency have been reported in middle-aged postmenopausal women. Interestingly, differences have not been found in attention, verbal fluency or memory when comparing cognitive function in late versus early postmenpausal stages. Cognitive decline associated with postmenopause may be due to several factors including hormonal changes, normal aging processes, age-related changes in dopaminergic neurotransmission and interindividual variations in brain function and cognitive abilities associated with genetic factors.

Chapter 3 - It has been observed that osteoarthritis is more prevalent once menopause is established, which has suggested the link between estrogens and healthy joints. In addition, deletion of estrogen receptors in female mice results in cartilage damage, osteophytosis and changes in subchondral bone of adult skeleton, suggesting that estrogen, through its receptor, has a protective role on the maintenance of normal joints. Furthermore, it has been postulated that acute loss of estrogens increases the levels of reactive oxygen species and activates nuclear factor-kB and cytokine production, which indicates that estrogens have also anti-inflammatory properties.

Pro-inflammatory cytokine expression has been shown to be attenuated by estrogen replacement. The ability of estrogen to attenuate the effects of oxidative stress is mediated, in part, by mechanisms that do not require stimulation of the nuclear-initiated actions of sex steroids. In spite of the negative effect of estrogen replacement reported in 2003 by the Women's Health Initiative (WHI) results, several studies published afterwards have explored the potential protective effect of estrogen supplementation in animal models and demonstrated possible reasons why these actions may justify a beneficial role of estrogens in degenerative joint disease.

In this chapter, we will revise the effects of estrogens in healthy and osteoarthritic or inflamed joints, especially in postmenopausal women.

Chapter 4 - Hepatocellular carcinoma (HCC) is one of the leading cancers in the world, which is an ultimate outcome of chronic hepatitis with persistent inflammation. Men have a higher incidence of HCC than women. Not only limited to the incidence, this sex difference is also reflected by the clinical course of disease progression and prognosis. The evidence from epidemiologic and animal studies suggested that this gender disparity might be caused by either the stimulatory effects of androgen and/or the protective effects of estrogen. The studies from the N'-N'-diethylnitrosamine (DEN) induced HCC mouse model provided a mechanism for the protective role of estrogen in female HCC. Estrogen was found able to protect hepatocytes from malignant transformation via down-regulation of the secretion of IL-6 from Kupffer cells, a critical process in this mouse model. Moreover, functioning as a strong endogenous antioxidant, estrogen can protect the hepatic steatosis and fibrosis in female livers, which are associated with the increased risk of HCC. It thus raised a unique function of estrogen axis in protecting hepatocarcinogenesis, which is in contrast to its tumor promoting roles in most other female cancers, such as breast cancer and ovarian cancer. Intriguingly, suppression of the ERα protein by overexpression of miR-18a, which occur preferentially in female HCC, was identified as a novel mechanism to block the tumor protective function of estrogen in female HCC. Several critical issues about the estrogen pathway in hepatocarcinogenesis still remained to be clarified, including the detail mechanisms underlying the tumor protective function of estrogen pathway in HCC, the key factor(s) involved in regulating the process, and also its interaction with the hepatitis viruses. Prospectively, the results can help design strategies by targeting to this estrogen axis for preventing or treatment of HCC.

Chapter 5 - Estrogens exert powerful effects on physiology by regulating gene expression. Their effects on the transcriptional activities of genes are well described in the literature. However, estrogens are also the hormones that are best known for post-transcriptional gene regulation. With the combination of transcriptional and post-transcriptional regulation, gene expression can be rapidly and powerfully controlled to maximize the utility of genomic information throughout the long lives of vertebrate animals. For some cell responses, up to 50% of the genes with altered expression are the result of changes in the stabilities of the messenger RNAs (mRNAs). For many genes including the estrogen receptor alpha (ER) gene, post-transcriptional regulation is the primary mode of alteration of expression. This indicates that post-transcriptional gene regulation is critical to estrogen actions because the ER protein determines the estrogen-responsiveness of animal tissues to a large extent. Estrogens have been shown to regulate the expression of certain genes by greatly altering the stabilities of mRNAs, including stabilizing ER mRNA. This effect may be ancient as it appears to be conserved from mammals to fish and frogs. Some studies have identified unique proteins that are induced by estrogens to bind and protect specific mRNAs from degradation. Recently, hundreds of microRNAs have been discovered and are estimated to actively regulate about one third of protein-encoding mRNAs. MicroRNAs associate with proteins in complexes on mRNAs, where they usually destabilize the mRNA or block its translation. Estrogens regulate the expression of microRNA genes in responsive tissues during normal physiology and disease processes. Other cell signals alter the expression of certain microRNAs that affect ER gene expression. Elucidation of the molecular mechanisms responsible for these post-transcriptional effects is certain to reveal novel molecular targets for therapeutic control of estrogen actions.

Chapter 1

ESTROGENS AS MEDIATORS OF OBESITY-INDUCED INFLAMMATION

Diana Teixeira, Diogo Pestana,
Conceição Calhau, and Rosário Monteiro

Department of Biochemistry, Faculty of Medicine,
University of Porto,
Alameda Professor Hernâni Monteiro,
Porto, Portugal

ABSTRACT

Obesity-related inflammation is a subject of great interest, not only for the exponential growth of obesity incidence but because obesity-driven inflammation may be an important instigator of the metabolic abnormalities that accompany the obese state. Estrogens have a role in metabolic control, through direct and indirect effects on the adipose tissue. The role of estrogens in inflammation and immune processes is now beginning to be unraveled with especial focus on cardiovascular and neurodegenerative disorders. In the case of the adipose tissue, effects of estrogens have remained rather unexploited regarding their possible association with the obese-related low-grade systemic inflammatory status. The adipose tissue is a source of estrogens and almost every cell type that composes it, including recruited inflammatory cells, may be a target for these hormones. In this regard, inflammatory cell recruitment into the adipose tissue in obese states has been considered central to the development the chronic inflammation associated with obesity. It has been suggested that subsets of infiltrating T cells may be a primary event in the initiation of adipose tissue inflammation. The recruitment of inflammatory cells to the site of inflammation is tightly governed by the expression of certain chemokines (e.g. MCP-1, MIP, RANTES) that play a central role in orchestrating the immune response. Therefore, inter-ference with chemokine expression by estrogens can substantially alter the quality of the immune response and its outcomes. On the other hand, the tissue environment may change the differentiation path engaged by recruited cells into different activation sates, often with almost opposing consequences. For example, macrophages may be classically (M1) or alternatively (M2) activated, expressing a pro- and anti-inflammatory cytokine profile, respectively. Also T lymphocytes display the same alternative activation. T_H1 cells secrete the cytokines IL-2, IL-12, interferon-gamma and TNFalpha, whereas T_H2 cells secrete the cytokines IL-4, IL-5, IL-10 and IL-13. The interference on this differ-entiation path by estrogens may therefore substantially alter the inflammatory response in the adipose tissue. Given the interplay of immune/inflammatory and metabolic processes in the adipose tissue, estrogens may interfere with the tissue's endocrine function, which can be reflected on plasmatic efferent messages and affect distant targets. Moreover, estrogens may change tissue composition in inflammatory cells for the upper-mentioned modulation of leukocyte recruitment and differentiation. In this line, it has been proposed that knowing the source of adipose tissue derived inflammation and inflammatory cell infiltration or understanding how these processes can be modulated may help develop therapeutic tools to hamper the metabolic dysfunction associated with obesity. Here, we propose the role that estrogens play in obesity related inflammation through effects on adipose tissue and circulatory inflammatory cell number, type and functional properties. We will start to briefly overview estrogen metabolism, handling and signaling in the adipose tissue and we will present evidence of estrogen modulation of the immune system that may reflect on, or that occur directly within the adipose tissue. Furthermore, we will highlight the interference of adipose tissue estrogen signaling by xenobiotics with estrogen modulating-properties and their potential to modulate immune/inflammatory processes based on the adipose tissue and possibly promote adipose tissue dysfunction.

Keywords: Adipose tissue, estrogens, inflammation, obesity

ABBREVIATIONS

αERKO, Estrogen receptor alpha knockout
17β-HSD, 17 beta-hydroxysteroid dehydrogenase
AF, Activation function
AKT, Alpha serine/threonine-protein kinase
AP, Activator protein
ArKO, Aromatase-knockout mouse
AT, Adipose tissue
ATM, Adipose tissue macrophage
BBP, Buthyl benzyl phthalate
Bcl, B-cell lymphoma
BMI, Body mass index
BPA, Bisphenol A
CCL, C-C motif ligand
CCR, C-C motif receptor
CREB, cAMP response element-binding
CYP450, Cytochrome P450
DDE, Dichlorodiphenyldichloroethylene
DDT, Dichlorodiphenyltrichloroethane
DES, Diethylstilbestrol
DHEA, Dehydroepiandrosterone
DHEAS, Dehydroepiandrosterone sulfate
ER, Estrogen receptor
ERK, Extracellular signal-regulated kinases
ERR, Estrogen-related receptors
FA, Fatty acid
FOX, Forkhead box proteins
FSH, Follicle-stimulating hormone
GPER, G protein-coupled estrogen receptor
GPR, G-protein-coupled receptor
HDL, High-density lipoprotein
HFD, High fat diet
ICAM-1, Intercellular adhesion molecule
IL, Interleukin
IL-1RA, IL-1 receptor antagonist
INF, Interferon
iNOS, Inducible nitric oxide synthase
JNK, c-jun kinase

MCP, Monocyte chemotactic protein
KO, Knockout
LBD, Ligand binding domain
LDL, Low-density lipoprotein
LPL, Lipoprotein lipase
LPS, Lipopolysaccharide
M1, Classically-activated macrophages
M2, Alternatively-activated macrophages
MAPK, Mitogen-activated protein kinase
MIP, Macrophage inflammatory protein
MMPs, Matrix metalloproteinases
ncmER, Non-classical membrane estrogen receptor
NF, Nuclear factor
NFAT, Nuclear factor of activated T-cells
NHANES, National Health and Nutrition Examination Survey
PCB, Polychlorinated biphenyl
PI3K, Phosphatidylinositol 3-kinases
PIP3, Phosphatidylinositol 3,4,5-trisphosphate
PBMC, Peripheral blood mononuclear cell
PPAR, Peroxisome proliferator-activated receptor
RANTES, Regulated on activation, normal T cell-expressed and secreted
ROS, Reactive oxygen species
SDF, Stromal cell-derived factor
SERM, Selective estrogen receptor modulators
SHBG, Sex hormone-binding globulin
SP, Specificity protein
TGF, Transforming growth factor
TIMP, Tissue inhibitor of metalloproteinases
TLR, Toll-like receptor
TNF, Tumor necrosis factor
UCP, Uncoupling protein
VCAM, Vascular cell adhesion molecule

ADIPOSE TISSUE-RELATED INFLAMMATION

Adipocyte size constitutes by itself a risk for inflammation. In fact, when the ability of expansion of the cells reaches the limit to accommodate the excess of nutrients, the diameter of adipocytes increases and they become a source of adipokines such as tumor necrosis factor (TNF)-α, interleukin (IL)-6 and monocyte chemotactic protein (MCP)-1, therefore consolidating the perpetuation of inflammation. Indeed, both in humans and in rodents, adipocyte size is a strong, direct predictor of macrophage accumulation in adipose tissue (AT) [1, 2]. During the development of obesity we can observe a dynamic change in the number of macrophages and also of their phenotype, in a way that mirrors the concept of T-cell activation [3, 4].

Macrophage infiltration was found to be higher in visceral compared with subcutaneous fat pads in a mouse model of obesity [3, 5]. Increased macrophage infiltration has also been reported in human visceral AT and is associated with clinical parameters of obesity co-morbidities. A positive correlation between adipocyte diameter and the number of infiltrating macrophages has also been found within each fat depot. However, omental adipocytes exhibit smaller adipose cell size. Therefore, adipocyte hypertrophy is not the sole determinant of macrophage recruitment to AT; it is also dependent on the anatomical location of the fat depot [6, 7].

Macrophages have a remarkable plasticity that allows them to efficiently respond to environmental signals. The local microenvironment may alter the pathway of cell differentiation by different activation stimuli, often with a nearly opposite outcome. For example, macrophages can be classically (M1) or alternatively (M2) activated, expressing a profile of pro- and anti-inflammatory cytokines, respectively. Stimulation of macrophages with T_H1 cytokines such as interferon (INF)-γ or bacterial byproducts, such as lipopoly-saccharide (LPS) promotes maturation of classically-activated macrophages (M1), which have a high inflammatory and bactericidal poten-tial, character-ized by the release of TNF-α and IL-6 and reactive oxygen species (ROS) production. However, TH2 cytokines, including IL-4 and IL-13, promote the alternative activation of macrophages (M2), which have high anti-parasitic capability and produce factors such as IL-10, IL-1 receptor antagonist (IL-1RA), arginase and transforming growth factor (TGF)-β. Moreover, M2 macrophages are involved in non-immunological processes, such as remodel-ing (repair) of AT and lipid metabolism [5, 6]. In several murine models fed a high fat diet (HFD) it was shown that newly recruited AT macrophages (ATM) were more pro-inflammatory than were the resident ATM in lean mice [8]. Further investigations in the same animals showed that newly AT-infiltrating macrophages are positive for the surface markers F4/80, CD11b and CD11c, and are preferentially recruited to clusters surrounding necrotic adipocytes while AT-resident macrophages are more interstitial, and express genes characteristics of the M2 activation state (Ym1, arginase 1 and IL-10) [9, 10].

Less information is available on the phenotype of ATM in humans. Boulier et al. [11], showed that native macrophages isolated from human AT express both M1 and M2 related markers, and the population of cells characterized by the expression of CD14 and CD206 (usually described on M2-activated/-resident anti-inflammatory macrophages) and the lack of CD16. Furthermore, with the increase in body mass index (BMI), human ATMs have a reduction of expression of several M1 markers and a concomitant increase in expression of M2 markers.

Natural killer cells also appear to contribute to AT inflammation [12]. These cells are an innate type of cytotoxic lymphocytes present in the stromal vascular fraction in the AT, forming a link between the innate and adaptive immune systems, and being increased in obesity [13]. The absence of natural killer cells in mice seems to protect them against diet-induced hyperglycemia and impairs the recruitment of macrophages to the AT. However, its stimulation leads to a reversed effect. These results, together with the knowledge that these cells infiltrate the AT in the late phases of obesity, provide evidence of their active role in AT inflammation and the development of morbidities associated with obesity [14].

Under normal conditions, cells involved in the adaptive immune system are present in the AT, where they play an important role in immune monitoring. In AT, the CD4$^+$ effector T cells can be classified into pro-inflammatory T_H1-polarized T cells (CD3$^+$), secreting IFN-γ and anti-inflammatory regulatory T_H2-polarized T cells, secreting IL-4 and IL-13. In mice, the T_H1- and T_H2-polarized T cells are predominantly in visceral AT, in comparison to the subcutaneous AT. However, diet-induced obesity leads to an increase in T_H1-polarized T cells, whereas the number of T_H2-polarized T cells remains static [14, 15].

In addition, animal studies denote that obesity leads to a significant decrease in regulatory T cell number, leading to insulin resistance and the increase in inflammatory markers in visceral the AT [16]. It was further observed that in the course of obesity there is an increase in CD8$^+$ effector T cells. The infiltration of effector T cells, also known as cytotoxic T cells, precedes the recruitment of macrophages to the AT. Depletion of effector T cells before inducing obesity in mice prevents M1 macrophage infiltration of the AT, without changing adiposity or the number of M2 macrophages and T_H1-polarized T resident cells. In obese mice with existing inflammation, the reduction of effector T cells mediated by antibodies, promotes glucose tolerance and insulin sensitivity and a concomitant decrease in AT inflame-mation, providing evidence for the role of these cells, not only in the initiation, but also preservation of inflammation in the AT. Despite this evidence substantiated in animal models, in humans more studies are needed to clarify the role of T cells in inflammation originating in the AT. Indeed, one study postulates clearly increased infiltration of lymphocytes in expanding AT, similarly to mice. The authors showed an increase in effector T cells and pro-inflammatory T_H1 polarized T cells in AT from obese subjects, the number of T cells in visceral AT being larger [17].

The recruitment of inflammatory cells into the site of inflammation is largely governed by the expression of certain chemokines (especially MCP-1, macrophage inflammatory protein-1 (MIP-1), regulated upon activation normal T-cell expressed and secreted (RANTES)/C-C motif ligand (CCL) 5 and stromal cells-derived factor 1 (SDF-1)) which play a central role in orchestrating the immune response in the AT [18, 19]. Additionally, studies suggest an increased CCL5 expression in the AT of obese subjects where it correlates with the amount of macrophages and inflammatory markers. Moreover, this chemokine protects macrophages from apoptosis and stimu-lates the transmigration and adhesion of blood monocytes through endothelial cells in the AT, perpetuating their survival and enabling the effective elimin-ation of nonviable adipocytes. Lymphocytes in the AT express C-C motif receptor (CCR) 6, the receptor for adipocyte-produced CCL20 chemokine, which seems to be an active participant in the cross-talk between lymphocytes and adipocytes in obesity [20].

Furthermore, nutrients like glucose and fatty acids (FA) seem to contri-bute to the recruitment of macrophages when in excess, regulating the expression of chemokines (MCP-1) by mechanisms involving the generation of ROS, the activation of nuclear factor (NF)-κB and peroxisome proliferator-activated receptor (PPAR)-γ. Free FA release from hypertrophied adipocytes can trigger pro-inflammatory responses in macrophages by acting on toll-like receptors (TLR) [21]. TLR4 knockout (KO) mice are partially protected from diet-induced insulin resistance, and are characterized by reduce AT and liver inflammation [22]. Additionally, the myeloid cell population characterized as $F4/80^+/CD11b^+/CD11c^+$ is more susceptible to free FA-mediated activation via TLR, compared with the $F4/80^+/CD11b^+/CD11c^-$ subpopulation [23]. This suggests that free FA, through the activation of TLR4 expressed on newly infiltrating ATM, promote the acquisition and/or maintenance of the inflammatory phenotype. Polyunsaturated FA and FA-derived molecules also bind the transcription factor PPAR-γ that is expressed in adipocytes as well as in macrophages. In the AT, induction of adipocyte differentiation by PPAR-γ is associated with the appearance of smaller adipocytes, which may partly account for the inhibitory effect of PPAR-γ on inflammatory gene expression [24]. PPAR-γ also appears to play a direct role in determining macrophage polarization in the AT, as its presence and/or activation are required for the expression of the alternatively M2-activated phenotype [25]. LPS-stimulated NF-κB signaling augments macrophage interference with adipocyte function and adipogenesis, which, reversely, is diminished by inhibition of NF-κB activation in macrophages cell lines [26]. Moreover, free FA, particularly saturated FA activate NF-κB via TLR4 in adipocytes and macrophages [27].

ESTROGEN SIGNALING

The classical nuclear estrogen receptor (ER) was cloned in 1985 [28, 29] and renamed ER-α. A second nuclear ER was discovered 10 years later, the ER-β [30]. The tissue distribution of ER-α and ER-β is different [31] and therefore it is expected that estrogens will have different effects in different tissues. ER-α is the predominant receptor in the bone, uterus, liver, and AT, whereas ER-β is the predominant receptor in the ovary and intestinal tract.

ER-α and ER-β belong to the steroid/thyroid hormone superfamily of nuclear receptors, members of which they share a common structure. They consist of three regions: the NH_2-terminal or A/B domain, the C or DNA-binding domain and the D/E/F domain or ligand-binding domain (LBD). The N-terminal A/B domain is the most variable region with < 20% amino acid identity between the two ERs and could confer subtype-specific actions and target genes. This region harbors the activation function (AF)-1 that is ligand independent and shows promoter- and cell-specific activity. The centrally located C-domain harbors the DNA binding domain, which is involved in DNA binding and receptor dimerization. This domain is highly conserved between ER-α and ER-β with 95% amino acid identity. The D-domain is referred to as the hinge domain and shows conservation between ER-α and ER-β (30%). This domain has been shown to contain a nuclear localization signal. The C-terminal E-domain constitutes the LBD and the two subtypes display 59% conservation in this region. The LBD contains a hormone-dependent AF-2 and is responsible for ligand binding and receptor dimerization. The F-domain has < 20% amino acid identity between the two ER subtypes and the functions of this domain are undefined [32-34]. In the absence of hormone, the receptor is sequestered within the nuclei of target cells in a multiprotein inhibitory complex. Binding of a ligand to the ERs triggers conformational changes in the receptor and this leads to a change in the rate of transcription of estrogen-regulated genes. These events comprise receptor dimerization, receptor-DNA interaction, recruitment of and interaction with coactivators and other transcription factors, and formation of a pre-initiation complex [35]. To modulate gene transcription, ERs recruit multiprotein complexes, containing chromatin-remodeling factors, histone acetyltransferases, histone deacetylases, proteosomal subunits and heat-shock proteins, to targets promoters [36]. Thus ERs can directly regulate many genes including those encoding hormones (e.g. oxytocin, angiotensinogen, prothymosin α), proteases (e.g. cathepsin D), angiogenesis promoters (e.g. vascular endothelial growth factor), cell survival proteins (e.g. Bcl-2) and cell proliferation proteins [37]. In addition to binding directly to DNA, 17β-estradiol-ER complexes can bind indirectly to chromatin via transcription factors such as activator protein (AP)-1 and NF-κB or can bind to DNA adjacent to transcription factors such as specificity protein (SP)-1 and forkhead box protein (FOX) A1, which stabilizes ER binding and promotes the assembly of transcriptional complexes [38]. ERs were also reported to regulate gene expression in a ligand independent manner, for instance by interacting with other nuclear hormones receptors, such as PPARs [39].

The recent development of KO mice lacking aromatase, ER-α or ER-β [40-43] and the identification of humans lacking aromatase or ER-α [44, 45] have allowed novel insights into the biological roles of estrogens, and ER-α or ER-β.

The third estrogen receptor, G-protein-coupled receptor 30 (GPR30), now known as G-protein-coupled ER (GPER), was identified in the late 1990's as an orphan 7-transmembrane domains G protein-coupled receptor with an intracellular localization [46] and on the plasma membrane [47], with low homology to existing G-protein-coupled receptors [48]. Unlike the classical ERs, GPER acts through a rapid non-genomic mechanism involving activation of the cAMP signaling pathways. Estradiol activates phosphoinositol 3-kinases (PI3K) through GPER. As a result of the accumulation of phosphatidylinositol 3,4,5-trisphosphate (PIP3), the anti-apoptotic and proliferative alpha serine/threonine-protein kinase (AKT) is activated. In 2000, Filardo et al. [49] demonstrated that the rapid activation of extracellular signal-regulated kinase (ERK) in breast cancer cells was dependent upon the presence of GPER.

Although the precise molecular mechanisms of nongenomic actions are not fully understood, it is known that some rapid estradiol effects can be initiated by ligand binding to membrane-associated ERs (mERs) that have been shown to be the same proteins as their nuclear receptor counterparts in several systems [50-52]. In addition to the classical genomic pathway, steroids can produce rapid (within a few minutes after application), nongenomic signaling effects via second messenger systems, for example, changes in Ca^{2+}, K^{+}, cAMP, and nitric oxide levels, activation of G protein-mediated events; and stimulation of different types of kinases such as extracellular-regulated kinases (Ras/Raf/MEK/ERK), PI3K, p38 mitogen-activated protein kinase (MAPK), and c-Jun kinase (JNK) [49, 53, 54]. Activation of MEK/ERK pathway consequently influences also gene expression profile through the activation of other transcriptional factors such as cAMP-related element binding (CREB) protein or nuclear factor of activated T-cells (NFAT) [55].

ER-α and ER-β are expressed in both subcutaneous and visceral ATs in human and rodents, which denotes that in AT estrogen signaling may occur through either of these ERs [56]. Furthermore, Dos Santos et al. [57] advocates that 17β-estradiol can act through membrane ER in adipocytes, to induce rapid effects through activation of MAPK, AP-1 and CREB protein. ERs are also expressed in preadipocytes [58] whereby estrogens can potentially regulate preadipocyte development and directly adipocytes. However, AT is much more than adipocytes. In fact, ER-α and ER-β are also expressed in other cell types found in AT, namely vascular endothelium, vascular smooth muscle and macrophages [59]. Thus, the effect of estrogens on AT must be viewed in light of a concerted action in all its different cell types.

Estrogen-related receptors (ERR) are a family of orphan receptors, which are closely related to ERs. The ERR family includes three members: ERR-α, ERR-β and ERR-γ. The three receptors are very similar and in terms of structure are very close to ERs. ERR are highly and rhythmically expressed in muscle, heart, bone and AT [60]. ERR-α is expressed throughout the adipocyte differentiation program [61] and in bone-derived macrophages activated by LPS or INF-γ [62]. It has been demonstrated that ERRs can interfere with estrogen signaling. Indeed ERs and ERRs recognize the same DNA-binding elements, share common target genes and are coexpressed in many tissues [60]. These receptors play a central role in regulating energy metabolism. ERR-α null mice are lean and resistant to HFD-induced obesity. One possible explanation for this effect is the fact that uncoupling protein (UCP)-1 expression is up regulated in ERR-α null mice white AT, a change that may contribute to an increase in energy expenditure and lower body weight [60].

It is interesting that when more than one ER is present in the same tissue or cell type for either genomic and nongenomic responses, ER-α tends to be driver of responses, while ER-β and GPER, when in the presence of ER-α, tend to antagonize its responses [63].

ESTROGEN TURNOVER IN THE ADIPOSE TISSUE

The influence of hormones on AT distribution appears to be related both to AT-specific expression of steroid hormone receptors and to local tissue steroid hormone metabolism. Moreover, AT is an important site for estrogen biosynthesis and storage. Although the gonads and the adrenal glands contribute to most of circulating sex hormones, AT, via enzyme activation and conversion, can contribute with up to 50% of circulating testosterone and around 100% of circulating estrogen in postmenopausal women [64, 65]. For example, AT aromatase converts androgens to estrogens: androstenedione to estrone and testosterone to estrogen. Additionally, AT 17beta-hydroxysteroid dehydrogenase (17β-HSD) converts weaker hormones to stronger ones: androstenedione to testosterone and estrone to estradiol. Subcutaneous AT expresses relatively more aromatase than 17β-HSD, whereas visceral AT expresses more 17β-HSD than aromatase. Therefore, higher visceral (central) adiposity may be associated with relatively more 17β-HSD expression, resulting in more local androgen production. Moreover, animals completely deficient in aromatase (ArKO) have been found to have increased visceral adiposity and insulin resistance [66]. Aromatase deficiency in men is associated with a disturbed lipid profile, and patients present BMI in the overweight range (25-30 kg/m^2), with accumulation of abdominal AT [67, 68]. Besides, circulating levels of triglycerides are generally elevated, with low circulating high-density lipoprotein (HDL) cholesterol. Significant aspects of aromatase deficiency, in both men and male mice, are reminiscent of the metabolic syndrome. The metabolic syndrome, can be considered a "constellation of closely related risk factors" for cardiometabolic events including abdominal obesity, insulin resistance, dyslipidemia (including elevated triglycerides and reduction of HDL cholesterol) and high blood pressure [69]. The loss of estrogens in men results in metabolic syndrome's key risk factors: truncal obesity, elevated blood lipids, fatty liver and severe insulin resistance, all characteristics matched in the aromatase deficient male mice, and clearly pointing to a significant relationship between estrogens and the metabolic syndrome in men [70].

MODELS OF ESTROGEN INSUFFICIENCY

Estrogen receptor α knockout mice (αERKO) display over 100% increase in AT compared with wild-type mice [71]. This increase is similar to those reported in ArKO [66] mice and in follicle-stimulating hormone (FSH) receptor KO mice [72] both of which have lack in 17β-estradiol. Thus, these results shows that loss of 17β-estradiol/ER-α signaling in αERKO mice, and lack of endogenous 17β-estradiol in ArKO and FSH receptor KO mice, which should lead to lack of signaling through ER-α and ER-β, led to similar increase in AT. Altogether, these results point toward the role of ER-α as the main regulator of estrogens' effects on the AT. Finally, removing the 17β-estradiol/ER-β signaling in αERKO mice by ovariectomy decreases body and fat-pad weights and adipocyte size. ER-β-mediated effects on AT are opposite to those of the ER-α. Although 17β-estradiol effects on AT are predominately through ER-α, ER-β may also be a player in the effect of estrogen on adipocytes [73]. Another investigation by Foryst-Luwig et al. [74] reveled that ER-β inhibited ligand-mediated transcriptional activity induced by PPAR-γ, resulting in a blockade of PPAR-γ-induced adipogenic gene expression and decreased adipogenesis.

Female and male αERKO mice are diabetes-prone and obese with several hepatic features of insulin resistance. On the other hand, ovariectomy on αERKO mice mice leads to normalized homeostasis of circulating glucose and insulin levels and reverses the obese phenotype, suggesting that ER-β-mediated estrogen activity may contribute to a diabetogenic and adipogenic phenotype. In contrast, ER-β knockout mice display improved insulin sensitivity and glucose tolerance without increased body fat content, suggesting that ER-α plays an important role in maintaining metabolic control [75].

Haas et al. [76], recently reported GPER expression in AT, and GPER-deficient mice generated by Wang et al. [77] are obese at 10-11 months of age. These data suggest that, in contrast to current concepts, estrogen-dependent signaling through GPER helps to counteract obesity development in a gender-independent fashion. These data are consistent with data from humans, where GPER has been detected in adipocytes [78]. Indirect evidence from studies using the selective estrogen receptor modulator raloxifene, suggests that GPER could be involved in adipocyte differentiation [79]. GPER deficient mice suffer from hyperglycemia, impaired glucose tolerance, and elevated blood pressure among other signs [80].

Strubbins et al. [81] have shown that male and female ovariectomized mice have larger adipocytes than non-ovariectomized female mice and female ovariectomized mice treated with 17β-estradiol when fed a HFD. An increase in adipocyte size can lead to a hypoxic environment which can worsen an already inflamed milieu. However, in contradiction, Rian et al. [82], showed that estradiol treatment of ovariectomized mice, despite improving insulin sensitivity and glucose tolerance, is associated with increased inflammation of AT, suggesting that estrogens contribute to (rather than attenuate) inflamemation.

The only clinical case of nonfunctional ER-α is a 28-year-old male patient who presented with glucose intolerance, hypoglycemia, obesity and hiperestrogenism [44]. Later, he developed premature coronary artery disease associated with low levels of total, HDL and LDL cholesterol [83]. Indeed, ER-α is now considered a candidate gene for obesity.

Genetic associations have been described for the ESR1 gene (coding for ER-α) and several pathological conditions related to metabolism, including cardiovascular disease, type two diabetes, myocardial infarction, hypertension and lipoprotein metabolism [84-86]. Polymorphisms in the ESR2 gene (coding for ER-β) have been associated with anorexia nervosa, bulimia nervosa, and premature coronary artery disease [87, 88]. A study in patients with coronary artery disease revealed that polymorphic changes in ER-β are linked to increased BMI, elevated triglycerides, and high apolipoprotein B concentrations. The authors propose that ER-β polymorphism is an independent risk factor for the disease [89].

Epidemiological studies show that premenopausal women are less likely to develop inflammation compared to age-matched men, suggesting a protective effect of estrogens against inflammation [90, 91]. Furthermore, postmenopausal women have a higher propensity for developing abdominal adiposity, which is associated with increase systemic levels of inflammatory cytokines, thus indicating that estrogens can modulate both body adiposity and systemic inflammation [92].

The lack of ovary-derived estrogens after menopause might play a part in increased adiposity, which in turn might enhance estrogen synthesis in the AT. Obese postmenopausal women have higher serum estrogen concentration than lean postmenopausal women [93]. Inflammatory cytokines such as TNF-α induce aromatase expression *in vitro* [94], so the inflammatory process probably leads to an increase in aromatase expression in different AT cell types (e.g. adipocytes, fibroblasts). On the other hand, estradiol has potent anti-inflammatory properties and suppresses the expression of IL-6 or TNF-α in macrophages and dendritic cells [28]. Hence, estrogens may have a paracrine role in AT inflammation targeted to alleviate potential tissue-damaging effects.

ESTROGENS AND ADIPOSE TISSUE MASS, DISTRIBUTION AND CELLULARITY

Important insights into the effects of estrogen on adipocyte development have come from *in vitro* and *in vivo* studies. In the 1970's, Roncari et al. [95], reported that 17β-estradiol stimulates proliferation of human preadipocytes. Similarly Dieudonné et al. [58] reported that 17β-estradiol stimulates proliferation of subcutaneous rat preadipocytes from females, but not males. The same phenomenon occurs in human-derived cells. According to Anderson et al. [96], 17β-estradiol may act as an important local factor influencing the proliferation of preadipocytes that may affect adipocyte number in a depot- and gender-specific manner in human abdominal subcutaneous and omental AT. Recent studies using both αERKO and ArKO mouse models have evidently pointed out that 17β-estradiol has an inhibitory effect on overall adipocyte number. Heine et al. [97] reported that both male and female αERKO mice have large increases in fat pad weight, which results from hyperplasia more than hypertrophy of adipocytes. Similar results were seen in ArKO mice [98]. Accordingly, the lack of estrogen signaling led to a large increase in the number of adipocytes, demonstrating that estrogen normally plays an inhibitory role during adipogenesis to limit adipocyte number.

Although AT mass is under genetic and environmental influences, women have a greater AT mass than men, a difference that appears at puberty, suggesting that sex steroids influence AT mass either directly or through other hormones such as growth hormone [99, 100]. Consistent with this finding is the sexual dimorphism in leptin production and secretion, a hormone which closely reflects total fat mass. Prior to puberty boys and girls have similar leptin levels. However, by late puberty leptin levels are significantly higher in females and remain higher in females through adulthood, supporting the observation that females have proportionally a greater fat mass [101, 102]. It is well recognized that estrogen influences body fat distribution by increasing gluteal and femoral fat content [99].

Concerning gender differences, adiponectin serum levels are moderately higher in women than men, and hormone replacement therapy does not affect adiponectin release in either pre- or postmenopausal women [103]. In this sense, gender differences in adiponectin appear to be due to a suppressive effect of androgens in men rather than a direct stimulation by estrogens [104]. There is no evidence of gender differences in circulating IL-6 or TNF-α levels in human [105].

Sex hormone-binding globulin (SHBG) is the major protein carrier of androgens and estrogens in the blood, and is reduced in states of increased abdominal obesity, namely visceral adiposity [106-108]. Its levels tend to be higher in women than men, likely due to the effects of higher estrogen concentration [106]. Therefore, increased SHBG levels in women compared with those of men may be related to the lower visceral AT accumulation observed in women.

Plasma levels of dehydroepiandrosterone (DHEA) and dehydroepian-drosterone sulfate (DHEAS) have a negative association with total body fat, subcutaneous AT and particularly visceral AT [109, 110]. Gender differ-ences in DHEAS have been reported, with increases serum levels in men compared with women. Moreover, in studies performed *in vitro*, DHEAS increases lipolysis in subcutaneous AT obteined from women after 2 hours, whereas in men lipolysis occurs preferentially in visceral AT but only after 24 hours. In AT cultures, DHEA inhibits adipocyte development and differentiation [110].

Concerning caloric intake, in the cohort of subjects from National Health and Nutrition Examination Survey (NHANES) III, men are reported to consume more calories compared with women despite the energy density of the calories consumed being the same between groups. This difference can be explained because of the greatest fat free mass in men and therefore higher required more energy levels [111]. Therefore, these findings indicate that women are consuming fewer calories for their body size than men; however they are storing energy in the form of fat at a much greater rate. Estrogens could influence the dietary intake of fat or alter the storage of fat through direct metabolic actions on lipolysis or decrease the oxidation of fatty acids leading to an accumulation of triglycerides in the AT. There is little evidence on the effect of estrogens on dietary intake of fat in women, however energy intake varies along then menstrual cycle [112]. An increase in fat or caloric intake is not likely to account for the gender differences in body fat since estroges have a negative effect on feeding through actions on the hypo-thalamus [113]. When ovariectomized and sham-operated rats were pair-fed, the weight compared to the shams, even in the absence of hyperphagia. This finding suggests that despite the estrogen effect on food consumption, the central effects of estrogen related to decreasing AT deposition might not entirely occur through decreases in energy intake. One explanation may be their effects on voluntary activity and energy expenditure, both of which are increased by estrogens [71]. In addition to its direct effect on the hypothalamus, estrogen may also regulate the production or response to adipose hormones such as leptin and affect processes such as food consumption and energy metabolism. Another mechanism through which estrogens decrease eating, at least in rats, is by increasing the satiating action of cholecystokinin [114].

In several mammals and women, higher levels of estrogens during the estrus and menstrual cycles and pregnancy lead to decreased food intake and fat accumulation [115]. In contrast ovariectomy, anti-estrogen treatment and menopause lead to an increase in food intake and meal size, effects that are reversed by 17β-estradiol replacement [35, 116]. These observations point toward the anorexigenic function of central action of estrogens. ER-α and ER-β are expressed in in several hypothalamic nuclei, and it seems that the central actions on 17β-estradiol on metabolism involve changes of feeding behavior rather than modulation of catabolism/anabolism of carbohydrates and lipids [117]. Silencing of ER-α in the ventromedial hypothalamus by RNA interference leads to adipocytes hyperplasia, obesity, decreased glucose tolerance and reduced energy expenditure [118]. The role of ER-β in the central regulation of feeding is less known. In ovariectomized rats there is increased food intake, body weight and abdominal fat accumulation, which can be reversed by 17β-estradiol. Nevertheless, administration of intracerebro-ventricular 17β-estradiol together with ER-β antisense oligodeoxynucleotides abrogates the anorexigenic effects of 17β-estradiol. This suggests that the central anorexigenic effects of 17β-estradiol may also occur via ER-β [119].

The increase in AT mass in women results from increases in adipocyte number as well as adipocyte size. Chumlea et al. revealed that adipocyte number in subcutaneous (gluteal) AT was increased by 34% in girls compared to boys at adolescence. Adipocyte size was also increased 45% compared to similar-aged boys [120]. Increased overall AT mass in women also partially reflects a greater number of adipocytes compared to men [121]. This points towards a role of estrogens in adipocyte development and establishment of adult adipocyte number, as well as in the modulation of adipocyte size in adult females. Nevertheless, AT deposition may also be modulated by other hormones (androgens), which clearly indicates that the sexual dimorphism in adipocyte number and size may not solely reflect estrogens effects in men *versus* women [122].

Estrogens can directly inhibit AT deposition by decreasing lipogenesis. This effect results mainly from decreasing activity of lipoprotein lipase (LPL), an enzyme that regulates lipid uptake by adipocytes. Ovariectomy increases LPL and lipid deposition in adipocytes and administering physiological doses of 17β-estradiol reverses this increase [123]. On the other hand, 17β-estradiol can indirectly affect lipolysis by inducing the lipolytic enzyme hormone-sensitive lipase [124] or by increasing the lipolytic effects of epinephrine [125]. Moreover fatty acid oxidation might also be increased, which might contribute to the decrease in AT mass induced by 17β-estradiol. However, contrary to its antilipogenic and lipolytic effect, estrogen attenuates the effect of α_{2A}- adrenergic receptors in human subcutaneous AT and decreases lipolysis. This effect could in part account for the increase deposition of subcutaneous AT in women compared to men [126].

ESTROGENS AND AT INFLAMMATION

Suppression of inflammatory responses represents a promising strategy to combat obesity associated disorders. Recent studies establish the mechanistic potential for estrogens to affect the inflammatory process. ER-α and, in some cases, ER-β are present in frontline immune and cytokine-producing cells, such as monocytes and macrophages, and estrogens activate these cells [127, 128]. Female rats and mice are relatively protected from HFD-induced obesity, insulin resistance and inflammatory responses [33]. Recent studies have shown that 17β-estradiol may play a role in reducing the inflammatory response in AT and cardiovascular and neural systems [129]. Some explanations for this have been shown using *in vivo* experiments. Vegeto et al. [127] have demonstrated that 17β-estradiol-activated ER-α decreases the number of pro-inflammatory cytokines. These anti-inflammatory properties can be partially explained by the ability of ERs to act as transcriptional repressors by inhibiting the activity of NF-κB [130]. However the estrogens' inhibitory effect on NF-κB is not fully understood. On the other hand, the PI3K pathway can be also implicated in the anti-inflammatory effects of estrogens. Ghisletti et al. [131] revealed that 17β-estradiol blocks LPS-induced NF-κB nuclear translocation in macrophages, an effect that involves the activation of PI3K.

Both human monocytes and macrophages express ER-α and ER-β. ER-α is the predominant receptor in macrophages and is up-regulated by estrogens (in macrophages but not in monocytes), whereas ER-β is the predominant receptor in monocytes and is unaltered by estrogens in either cell type [132]. GPER is highly expressed in human macrophages [133]. The roles of estrogens in the macrophage-related inflammation are complex. In mice, estrogens inhibit LPS-induced mouse homologue of MCP-1 in peritoneal macrophages as well as IL-6, IL-1 and TNF-α in splenic macrophages [134, 135]. Recent evidence suggests that activation of GPER participates in the down-regulation of TNF-α and IL-6 in human macrophages [133].

Estrogens have been reported to have anti-inflammatory properties [136]. Arenas et al. [137], found that circulating levels of TNF-α were 7-fold higher in ovariectomized rats compared with estrogen-replaced ovariectomized rats or those with estrogen production. Human studies have also noted that menopause is associated with increased cytokine levels, including TNF-α, IL-1 and IL-6, these levels being substantially lower in women receiving hormone replacement therapy [138]. In an extensive review, Straub [28] suggests that physiological levels of estrogens and estrogens levels attained during pregnancy and the hormone therapy inhibit secretion of pro-inflammatory cytokines, namely TNF-α, IL1-β, IL-6, MCP-1, inducible nitric oxide synthase (iNOS) and matrix metalloproteinases (MMP) and stimulate the synthesis and secretion of anti-inflammatory cytokines such as IL-4, IL-10, TGF-β, tissue inhibitor of metalloproteinases (TIMP) and osteoprotegerin. These effects are mediated predominantly through ER-α signaling mechanisms in otherwise unstimulated cells. In contrast, with decreases in 17β-estradiol concentration at menopause, secretion of pro-inflammatory cytokines increases as does the expression of cellular surface adhesion molecules (E-selectin, vascular cell adhesion molecule (VCAM)-1 and intracellular adhesion molecule (ICAM)-1). All of these responses are reverted with the restoration of the levels of estrogens to those of premenopause.

The advent of molecular biology techniques has allowed a perspective on the biology of AT in the context of obesity. Knowledge of the AT transcriptome of obese subjects before and after weight loss showed an increase of genes related to extracellular matrix components, and an increase in AT fibrosis [14]. Additionally, an analysis of AT biopsies transcriptome from healthy individuals before and after stimulation with LPS showed changes in the AT after induction of acute inflammation [139]. Thus, differences were found in the inflammatory state, in the expression of multiple molecules belonging to the secretome of adipocytes (particularly adipokines) and monocytes (chemokines involved in the recruitment and activation of immune cells), adhesion molecules and antioxidant molecules [14, 28]. The function of some of the genes described is still unknown, and may enclose new mechanisms involved on AT inflammation, potential biomarkers or therapeutic targets for diseases associated with obesity.

Plasma levels of MCP-1 have been reported to be lower in postmen-pausal women receiving hormone replacement therapy compared to those not receiving hormone replacement therapy [140]. Treatment with 17β-estradiol has been reported to inhibit LPS-induced MCP-1 mRNA expression in macrophage cell lines [135].

In human peripheral blood mononuclear cells (PBMCs), in the presence of LPS (as cell/activator/stimulator substance), 17β-estradiol inhibited TNF-α at concentrations of 10^{-10} to 10^{-7} M in male subjects and at 10^{-8} to 10^{-7} M in female subjects. However, 17β-estradiol had a stimulating effect in the absence of LPS [105]. In human whole blood cultures, 17β-estradiol at 10^{-10} to 10^{-8} M decreased spontaneous secretion of IL-6, TNF-α, IL-1RA, IL-1β and the ratio of IL-1β/IL-1RA compared with control, but 17β-estradiol did not strongly change LPS-stimulated cytokine secretion [141].

XENOESTROGENS AND OBESITY-ASSOCIATED COMPLICATIONS

The causes of the growing prevalence of obesity are a major challenge for medical and scientific community. Accumulating data suggest an important role for toxicology of obesity [142]. In 2002, Baillie-Hamilton [143] proposes a provocative hypothesis to explain the global obesity epidemic. The author emphasized the fact that the current exponential increase of obesity could not be justified merely by the alterations of food intake and a lack of physical activity. At the same time, other authors claimed that genetic predisposition could be a major component resulting in obesity [144]. Nevertheless, Baillie-Hamilton upraised the objection that the human genome cannot have undergone particularly important mutations over the last decades, and underlined that the correlation between enhanced accumulation of environmental industrial chemicals and increase of obesity incidence might not be a simple coincidence.

Nowadays, there are several lines of evidence that highlight the potential involvement of environmental "obesogens" [143, 145-147] which can be defined functionally as xenobiotic chemical agents that can disrupt the normal development and homeostatic control of adipogenesis and energy balance [148].

Xenoestrogens also termed estrogen disruptors are man-made chemicals produced by industry and released into the environment, namely, phthalate or bisphenol A (BPA) plasticizers, organotins, pesticides, dioxins, poly-chlorinated biphenyls (PCB), flame retardants, or alkylphenols. Some naturally- occurring xenoestrogens can also be found in plants or fungi, such as the so-called phytoestrogens: genistein, daidzein or the mycoestrogen zearalenone. Such estrogen mimetics were noted for their effect on wildlife in the 1960´s when naturalists such as Rachel Carson drew attention to the endocrine-disrupting effects of some pesticides (notably dichlorodiphenyl-trichloroethane (DDT) [149]). These compounds have in common lipophilic phenolic rings and other hydrophobic components, a characteristic they share with steroid hormones and related nuclear receptor-activating compounds. They also exhibit potent lipophilic, fat-soluble and long half-life properties [150].

For many years the mechanisms via which many xenoestrogens acted remained a mystery. This lack of a mechanistic explanation existed because, while these compounds can affect animal functions and development at relatively low concentrations, experimental systems for testing the classical nuclear transcriptional activities of xenoestrogens showed weak or no activity [151, 152]. Nevertheless, some mechanisms have been unraveled. These compounds may act as inappropriate estrogens, and/or can interfere with endogenous estrogen actions.

The action of xenoestrogens can be mediated by two mechanisms, either they temporarily or permanently alter the feedback loops in the brain, pituitary, gonads, thyroid, and other components of the endocrine system by mimicking the effects of estrogens and triggering their specific receptors or they bind to hormone receptors and block the action of natural hormones. They also interfere with the metabolism, production, transport and action of these endogenous hormones [32, 153]. The structural similarities between xenoestrogens and endogenous estrogen allow binding to ERs and activation in the absence of the endogenous, or natural estrogen. Their hydrocarbon structures and halide contens may be a factor as to the why they can bind to the two nuclear receptors. Estrogen and estrogen-like chemicals bind at the LBD and demonstrate different binding modes. ER consists of three-layered antiparallel alpha-helical, which consists of a central core consisting of three helices (H5/6, H9, H10) and an additional layer on the top and bottom with helices (H1-4 and H7, H8, H11). This arrangement creates a groove for ligand binding [154]. Estrogen binds diagonally across the cavity between H11, H13 and H6. This arrangement gives it a low-energy conformation. Recent studies have shown that xenoestrogens possess similar binding affinities to ER when compared natural or endogenous estrogen and this is mainly due to an overall ring structure which is preferred during ER binding. Not only do xenoestrogens bind to ER but these molecules may also have higher affinity for ER than endogenous estrogens [155].

Environmental estrogens produce potent membrane-initiated signaling effects similar but not identical to those elicited by 17β-estradiol. There is a paucity of data that on the ability of environmental estrogens to mediate nongenomic effects at low concentrations. However, there are few data [156-160] addressing the ability of environmental estrogens to mediate nongenomic estrogenic actions, and many studies on this phenomenon have used concentrations of xenoestrogens much higher than those that found in contamination sites.

Watson et al. [161] postulated that environmental estrogens could initiate their actions from the plasma membrane. Further research about the role of ER-α at the membrane has described that xenoestrogens induce ERK-1 and ERK-2, although their responses are different depending on the xenoestrogens being tested [162, 163]. Thus endosulfan, nonylphenol, dicholorodiethyl-dochloroethylene (DDE), dieldrin and coumestrol phosphorylate ERK with a unique pattern at low concentrations (in the nanomolar range). Other rapid actions of xenoestrogens are mediated by receptors different from the classical ER-α and ER-β. In fact DDE, binds GPER and activates adenylyl cyclase increasing cAMP production [164]. The ncmER may be another target for xenoestrogens. In insulin-releasing β-cells and glucagon-releasing α-cells, there are ncmER that mediate the actions of 17β-estradiol, BPA and diethylstilbesterol (DES). In β-cells this receptor regulates Ca^{2+} signals at low concentrations of BPA and this action is involved in the activation of the transcriptional factor CREB [165]. Xenoestrogens also rapidly modify other signaling pathways. Therefore 25 μM of DES, BPA and 10 μg/mL of PCB change the phosphorylation state of proteins belonging to the large family of MAPK in mussel hemocytes [166].

Xenoestrogens may also have effects on estrogen metabolism in a number of ways. Some can alter serum lipid concentration, ultimately enhancing the production of 17β-estradiol and other steroids. Furthermore, some xeno-estrogens can alter metabolic enzymes that are necessary for converting cholesterol to steroid hormones. Numerous xenoestrogens can activate P450 cytochromes (CYP450), which are involved in the metabolism of most steroid hormones and xenoestrogens [167]. They have been shown to up-regulate CYP450 aromatase expression, and act as an initiator of significantly raised intracellular estradiol production in adipose cells [142]. As adipogenesis increases under the action of up-regulated P450 aromatase and raised intracellular estradiol, the adipocyte releases increasing quantities of leptin and free FA that activate NF-κB in adjacent macrophages, which further upregulate aromatase via cyclooxygenase-2/prostaglandin E2, IL-1β and TNF-α [21].

Plants produce a wide variety of secondary metabolites some of which are phytoestrogens, chemicals that have similar structures as 17β-estradiol and display estrogenic activity through ER signaling pathways. The best studied are phytoestrogens, which include isoflavones, lignans and coumestans and stilbenes [168]. Phytoestrogens are present in common foods such as soybeans, grains, fruits and vegetables [169]. Phytoestrogens can bind to both ER-α and ER-β. However, they appear to have higher affinity for ER-β. In fact, this affinity may be dose-dependent but, generally, phytoestrogens have lower affinity to the ERs than estradiol [168].

It has been reported that isoflavones, nonsteroidal diphenolic compounds with a structure closely resembling the steroid structure, have both agonistic and antagonistic effects, though they are strong ER-β and weak ER-α agonists [168]. Isoflavones, such as daidzein and genistein, are two of the most abundant phytoestrogens in the human diet and are selective estrogen receptor modulators or biochemical compounds that are able to activate or antagonize ER [170].

The isoflavone genistein appears to be one significant regulator of adipocyte metabolism. A recent study showed that genistein at pharmacologically high doses did indeed inhibited AT fat deposition, while at low doses, similar to those found in Western and Eastern diets, in soy milk or in food supplements containing soy, it induced AT deposition, especially in males [171]. It exhibits a hypolipidemic effect by inhibiting the adipocyte maturation. *In vitro* studies demonstrate that genistein decreases insulin-induced lipogenesis in a primary culture of rat adipocytes and preconfluent and postconfluent 3T3-L1 preadipocyte cell line. Additionally genistein decreases adipocyte number and lipid filling in primary bone marrow stromal cells or it inhibits differentiation of preadipocytes from human subcutaneous AT [172-175]. Most animal models used to elucidate the effects of isoflavones on obesity are rodent strains with either genetically or diet-induced obesity. Ovariectomy of females is also a common tool, as removal of the ovaries causes increases in AT similar to the increases seen in women after menopause

[176]. From experiments on animal models, many exciting results of the effects of dietary isoflavones have been obtained. These *in vivo* experiments have established that the reduction effects of isoflavones on AT, as shown *in vitro*, are not simply reflected in a decrease in body weight *in vivo*. There is some controversy, and many contradictory reports about the effect of isoflavones in food intake. Wade et al. [177] reported that isoflavones increase food and water intake, whereas others studies have shown that isoflavones decrease food intake [171, 178]. However, three soy isoflavones - genistein, daidzein and glycitein - have been demonstrated to affect AT without affecting food consumption. Thereafter, Kim et al. [179] showed that a diet containing 1500 mg genistein per kilogram of diet fed to 9 month-old ovariectomized mice for 3 weeks decreases body weight by 9% and decreased parametrial fat pad and inguinal fat pad weights by 22% and 19%, respectively. This suggests that a distinction between fat pad weight and body weight is important when considering whether isoflavones could potentially be used for weight reduction in humans, because these factors do not necessarily correlate. Corroborating this, Naaz et al. [180] reported that levels of 500 to 1500 mg genistein per kilogram of diet fed to 25 to 27 day-old ovariectomized mice for 12 days decreased parametrial and inguinal fat pad weights by 37% to 57%. The great difference in the level of weight reduction between the two groups the two experiments may be ascribed to a lower responsiveness of older mice to genistein that was due to reduced sensitivity of ER. In fact, the important role of the ER in the effect of genistein was supported when genistein failed to reduce adipose weight in αERKO. In 2006, Penza et al. [171] suggested that the antilipogenic action of genistein and downregulation of adipogenic genes require the expression of ER-β. All together these results point out that the interaction and cooperation between ER-α and ER-β in the downregulation of estrogen-dependent genes is crutial for the regulation of AT.

The reduction of AT by isoflavones *in vivo* seems to be mediated by adipocyte apoptosis and reduction of individual adipocyte size. Indeed, Kim et al. [179] reported that a dose of 1500 mg genistein per kilogram of diet increases DNA fragmentation in inguinal fat pad by 290% in ovariectomized adult mice, a result that confirms that adipose apoptosis contributes to the genistein-mediated reduction of AT. However, DNA fragmentation was not detected in retroperitoneal and parametrial fat pads what suggests that apoptosis by genistein may be fat depot-specific. Furthermore, Naaz et al. [180] stated that genistein leads to a decrease in adipocyte size in juvenile ovariectomized mice, caused at least in part by decreases in LPL mRNA in AT. Thus, similar to the effects of estrogen, the effects of genistein on AT could due to an inhibition of lipogenic LPL that regulates adipocyte lipid uptake.

While there are many studies on isoflavones, there are significantly fewer studies on coumestans and stilbenes. Coumestans are potent activators of the ER signaling pathway but are not as prevalent in the diet. Resveratrol is the most common stilbene and its use as a chemopreventive agent against breast cancer is actively being studied in rodent models [181].

On the other hand, phytoestrogens have been noted to be inhibitors of enzymes involved in the synthesis of estrogens. Concerning genistein, in addition to tyrosine kinase, it inhibits enzymes like DNA topoisomerases I e II, 5 α-redutase, aromatase, mitogen-activated protein kinases and protein histidine kinase activity [182]. This, in turn, leads to a decreased in circulating levels of free estrogen and less peripheral conversion of androgens to estrogens.

The phenolic isoflavone phytoestrogen genistein, displays high binding affinity and selectivity for ER-β but also demonstrates significant binding and activity towards GPER [183, 184].

Epidemiological studies have shown that exposure to xenoestrogens is near ubiquitous among humans. Wittassek et al. [185] showed that in a German sample, phthalates metabolites have been detected in 98% of urine samples, indicating ubiquitous exposure through the last 20 years. In another study, Calafat et al. [186] found that bisphenol A was detected in 95% of the 394 adults samples and 4-nonylphenol was detected in 51% of urinary samples. Organochlorine concentrations were also found in plasma and in abdominal and femoral subcutaneous AT among men in a weight loss program [187, 188]. However, there is a scarcity of population-based epidemiologic studies evaluating associations between xenoestrogens and obesity, and some controversy in the existing data. Goncharov et al. [189] studied the association between high serum PCBs and serum lipids in Native American population and showed that individuals with higher levels of PCBs tend to have higher levels of total serum lipids, showing a significant association among PCBs, lipids, age and BMI. Contrarily, Hue et al had not found an association between total plasma organochlorine concentration and BMI in 53 individuals ranging from lean to obese. Nevertheless, Pelletier et al. [190] revealed that plasma organochlorine concentrations were positively associated with higher BMI and fat mass in humans. Another study showed that serum BPA was detected to be higher in non-obese and obese women with polycystic ovary syndrome compared with BPA levels in non-obese normal women [191]. In a population of the NHANES an association between persistent organic pollutants (polychlorinated dibenzo-p-dioxins, and organochlorine pesticides) and diabetes has found among obese individuals compared to lean individuals [192]. Further investigations showed the inverse association of non-dioxin PCBs with BMI and a positive association between organochlorine pesticides and BMI [193, 194]. Taken together, these epidemiological reports suggest that environmental exposures to various xenoestrogens play a role in over-weight/obesity and comorbidities. Since there are so many diverse chemicals involved, they are most likely exerting their effects through multiple pathways.

Recently, a new target of xenoestrogens has been proposed, the adipocyte. A newly emerging hypothesis is that exposure to environmental chemicals during development may play a role in the development of obesity in life [143]. One example is octylphenol, a chemical widely used as surfactant, which can up regulate resistin, an adipocyte specific hormone that may cause insulin-resistance and decrease adipocyte differentiation [194]. Other example are brominated flame retardants a group of industrial chemicals produced in high quantities, highly lipophilic and that bioaccumulate in AT [153]. Bisphenol A is a high production volume chemical used in the manufacture of polycarbonate plastics, which can be used in baby and water bottles, and epoxide resins that are used in food container linings, whereby the dietary ingestion is considered the primary source of general population exposure [195]. Studies on the impact of BPA on AT yielded conflicting results, most likely due to the wide range of administered doses. Thus, concerning BPA accumulation in rat AT was low in one study [196] but higher in another [197]. The time of exposure is important too. When given the rats at higher doses for 15 days, BPA causes reduction in body weight and a lower feeding efficiency [198], while others found that feeding BPA to rats for three months did not alter body weight, fat depots or triglyceride levels. *In vitro* studies provide further evidence for the role of BPA in AT development. Thus, BPA lead to an increase in 3T3-L1 differentiation and BPA in combination with insulin accelerate adipocyte formation [199, 200]. Recently, Hugo et al. [78] reported that BPA at low environmental-relevant doses of BPA have also been reported to inhibit adiponectin synthesis and to stimulate the release of inflammatory adipokines such as IL-6 and TNF-α from human AT, suggesting that BPA is involved in inflammatory state associated with obesity.

Gesta et al. [201], point toward a role of developmental genes in the origin of obesity and body fat distribution. Thus the exposure to environmental chemicals with hormonal activity may be altering gene expression involved in programming adipocytes. Several genes have been implicated in altering adipocyte distribution and function such as *Hoxa5*, *Gpc4*, and *Tbx15* and adipocyte distribution such as such as *Thbd*, *Nr2f1* and *Sfrp2*. Newbold et al. [202] investigated the effect of DES in these target genes by microarrays analysis in uterine samples from DES-treated mice compared with controls at 19 days of age. These authors showed that genes involved in adipocyte distribution were not altered in the uterus following neonatal DES exposure, however genes involved in fat distribution were. *Thbd* and *Nr2f1* were significant downregulated and *Sfrp2* was significantly upregulated in DES-treated mice. These findings support the idea that environmental estrogen may play a role in regulating the expression of obesity-related genes during development.

There is widespread acceptance of the developmental origins hypothesis, which suggests that action of a stimulus during a specific critical period *in utero* or early postnatal development can lead to programmed alterations in tissue structure and function, predisposing the individual to later disease. Therefore, obesity and metabolic disorders in adult may represent a complex interaction between early developmental influences on the disease suscep-tibility and later lifestyle, which builds on the level of predisposition, thus more of a "lifetime" than simply a "lifestyle" disorder. An obvious question is whether other changes to our environment (or lifestyles) might impact on our predisposition to disease, and whether this might contribute to the recent obesity epidemic. Several studies have been reported that exposure to xeno-estrogens, including phytoestrogens, synthetic estrogens (e.g. DES) and environmental xenoestrogens causes changes in body weight and development of obesity: developmental exposure to DES is associated with decreased body weight gain [203, 204]; neonatal exposure to soybean products enriched in phytoestrogens altered body weight, adiposity and adipokines in adult female, indicating that exposure to phytoestrogens early in life affects mouse white AT; a significant decrease in maternal body weight gain and food consumption was seen in pregnant rats treated with BBP on days 15 and 17 of pregnancy. This treatment also caused significant decrease in weights of *fetus* [205]. Rubin et al. [206], showed that the offspring of female rats exposed perinatally to low doses of BPA, from day 6 of pregnancy through the period of lactation, exhibited an increased body weight that was apparent soon after birth and continued into adulthood. Some authors have observed a low birth weight on rats exposed to PCBs measured in maternal serum, although no association between birth weight and maternal serum polybrominated biphenyls at conception or enrollment of PCBs in 444 mothers and their infants were observed in another study [207, 208]. However, the cellular and molecular mechanism by which xenoestrogens are involved in the regulation of body weight and obesity are poorly understood, pointing the urgency of a comprehensive investigation in this area. The concept of the "developmental origins of adult disease" [209], as the term implies, suggests that there is a time lag between exposure and manifestation of disease. In other words, the effects of exposure during development may not be readily apparent until much later life.

Transgenerational effects may also be seen following exposure to xenoestrogens during development, not only to the exposed individual but also to subsequent generations. This would imply that the mechanisms of transmission occur through the germ line and they may involve genetic and/or epigenetic events. Epigenetic programing plays an important role in an organism's reaction to environmental stresses during critical developmental periods [210]. Epigenetics literally means "above the genetics". In the case of epigenetic changes, effects are not due to a genetic impairment but to modifycations of factors that regulate gene expression such as DNA methylation and histone acetylation. Although our genetic code is relatively static throughout our lives, our epigenetic code must change dramatically during development to initiate differential gene expression amongst developing tissues. Thus far, xenoestrogens studies have mainly focused on epigenetics changes in reproductive tract tissues: *in utero* exposure of mice to DES has been shown to result in the hypermethylation of the developmentally critical (especially to uterine organogenesis) *Hoxa10* gene [211]. In addition, grandchildren of DES exposed women were reported to have higher incidences of rare reproductive disorders [212]. In agouti mice, Dolinoy et al. [213] showed that *in utero* BPA exposure decreases CpG methylation and that methyl-donor supplementation negated BPA-related hypomethylation. In human placental cell lines, BPA exposure has been shown to alter miRNA expression levels [214]. However, similar effects can conceivably occur in other differentiating endocrine responsive tissues.

Another key concept regarding the endocrine disruption is that there may be non-traditional dose response curves as an inverted "U" or even multiple "U" shaped curves, making it impossible to predict responses in the low dose environmental exposure range based on exposures in the low dose environmental range [215]. Although these concepts have been well documented for hormones and neurotransmitters, they are just starting to be appreciated for xenoestrogens.

CONCLUSION

There is a growing amount of evidence that estrogen signaling disruption plays a role in the metabolic and inflammatory disturbances that accompany the excess deposition of dysfunctional adipose tissue that occurs in obesity. However, a detailed description of the precise mechanisms related to estrogen insufficiency and or estrogen excess in obesity-related mechanisms is still far from being complete. Although the past years have been fruitful in such research, the advances made on the relationship between obesity-related inflammation and metabolic disturbances had left a blank on how these processes can be mediated by estrogens, either endogenously produced or xenoestrogens. It is therefore mandatory, that the association between estrogen signaling modulation and obesity-related inflammation are deeply investigated in the hope that it constitutes a therapeutic avenue to help counteract the wicked disorders that obesity causes.

ACKNOWLEDGMENTS

This work was supported by FCT (PEst-OE/SAU/UI0038/2011, SFRH/ BPD/40110/2007, SFRH/BD/46640/2008, SFRH/BD/64691/2009).

REFERENCES

[1]   Mosser DM. The many faces of macrophage activation. *J Leukoc Biol* 2003; 73:209-12.

[2]   Gordon S. Do macrophage innate immune receptors enhance atherogenesis? *Dev Cell* 2003; 5:666-8.

[3]   Weisberg SP, McCann D, Desai M, Rosenbaum M, Leibel RL, Ferrante AW, Jr. Obesity is associated with macrophage accumulation in adipose tissue. *J Clin Invest* 2003; 112:1796-808.

[4]   Xu H, Barnes GT, Yang Q, *et al.* Chronic inflammation in fat plays a crucial role in the development of obesity-related insulin resistance. *J Clin Invest* 2003; 112:1821-30.

[5]   Mantovani A, Sica A, Sozzani S, Allavena P, Vecchi A, Locati M. The chemokine system in diverse forms of macrophage activation and polarization. *Trends Immunol* 2004; 25:677-86.

[6]   Gordon S. Alternative activation of macrophages. *Nat Rev Immunol* 2003; 3:23-35.

[7]   Cancello R, Tordjman J, Poitou C, *et al.* Increased infiltration of macrophages in omental adipose tissue is associated with marked hepatic lesions in morbid human obesity. *Diabetes* 2006; 55:1554-61.

[8]   Lumeng CN, Deyoung SM, Bodzin JL, Saltiel AR. Increased inflammatory properties of adipose tissue macrophages recruited during diet-induced obesity. *Diabetes* 2007; 56:16-23.

[9]   Lumeng CN, DelProposto JB, Westcott DJ, Saltiel AR. Phenotypic switching of adipose tissue macrophages with obesity is generated by spatiotemporal differences in macrophage subtypes. *Diabetes* 2008; 57:3239-46.

[10]   Murdoch C, Muthana M, Lewis CE. Hypoxia regulates macrophage functions in inflammation. *J Immunol* 2005; 175:6257-63.

[11]   Bourlier V, Zakaroff-Girard A, Miranville A, *et al.* Remodeling phenotype of human subcutaneous adipose tissue macrophages. *Circulation* 2008; 117:806-15.

[12]   Ohmura K, Ishimori N, Ohmura Y, *et al.* Natural killer T cells are involved in adipose tissues inflammation and glucose intolerance in diet-induced obese mice. *Arterioscler Thromb Vasc Biol* 2010; 30:193-9.

[13]   Caspar-Bauguil S, Cousin B, Galinier A, *et al.* Adipose tissues as an ancestral immune organ: site-specific change in obesity. *FEBS Lett* 2005; 579:3487-92.

[14]   Sell H, Eckel J. Adipose tissue inflammation: novel insight into the role of macrophages and lymphocytes. *Curr Opin Clin Nutr Metab Care* 2010; 13:366-70.

[15]   Winer S, Paltser G, Chan Y, *et al.* Obesity predisposes to Th17 bias. *Eur J Immunol* 2009; 39:2629-35.

[16]   Feuerer M, Herrero L, Cipolletta D, *et al.* Lean, but not obese, fat is enriched for a unique population of regulatory T cells that affect metabolic parameters. *Nat Med* 2009; 15:930-9.

[17]   Duffaut C, Galitzky J, Lafontan M, Bouloumie A. Unexpected trafficking of immune cells within the adipose tissue during the onset of obesity. *Biochem Biophys Res Commun* 2009; 384:482-5.

[18]   Kintscher U, Hartge M, Hess K, *et al.* T-lymphocyte infiltration in visceral adipose tissue - A primary event in adipose tissue inflammation and the development of obesity-mediated insulin resistance. *Arteriosclerosis Thrombosis and Vascular Biology* 2008; 28:1304-10.

[19]   Keophiphath M, Rouault C, Divoux A, Clement K, Lacasa D. CCL5 Promotes Macrophage Recruitment and Survival in Human Adipose Tissue. *Arteriosclerosis Thrombosis and Vascular Biology* 2010; 30:39-U113.

[20]   Duffaut C, Zakaroff-Girard A, Bourlier V, *et al.* Interplay between human adipocytes and T lymphocytes in obesity: CCL20 as an adipochemokine and T lymphocytes as lipogenic modulators. *Arterioscler Thromb Vasc Biol* 2009; 29:1608-14.

[21]   Suganami T, Nishida J, Ogawa Y. A paracrine loop between adipocytes and macrophages aggravates inflammatory changes: role of free fatty acids and tumor necrosis factor alpha. *Arterioscler Thromb Vasc Biol* 2005; 25:2062-8.

[22]   Shi H, Kokoeva MV, Inouye K, Tzameli I, Yin H, Flier JS. TLR4 links innate immunity and fatty acid-induced insulin resistance. *Journal of Clinical Investigation* 2006; 116:3015-25.

[23]   Nguyen MT, Favelyukis S, Nguyen AK, *et al.* A subpopulation of macrophages infiltrates hypertrophic adipose tissue and is activated by free fatty acids via Toll-like receptors 2 and 4 and JNK-dependent pathways. *Journal of Biological Chemistry* 2007; 282:35279-92.

[24]   Jernas M, Palming J, Sjoholm K, *et al.* Separation of human adipocytes by size: hypertrophic fat cells display distinct gene expression. *FASEB J* 2006; 20:1540-2.

[25]   Stienstra R, Duval C, Keshtkar S, van der Laak J, Kersten S, Muller M. Peroxisome proliferator-activated receptor gamma activation promotes infiltration of alternatively activated macrophages into adipose tissue. *Journal of Biological Chemistry* 2008; 283:22620-7.

[26]   Lacasa D, Taleb S, Keophiphath M, Miranville A, Clement K. Macrophage-secreted factors impair human adipogenesis: involvement of proinflammatory state in preadipocytes. *Endocrinology* 2007; 148:868-77.

[27]   Lee JY, Hwang DH. The modulation of inflammatory gene expression by lipids: mediation through Toll-like receptors. *Mol Cells* 2006; 21:174-85.

[28]   Straub RH. The complex role of estrogens in inflammation. *Endocrine Reviews* 2007; 28:521-74.

[29] Green S, Kumar V, Krust A, Walter P, Chambon P. Structural and functional domains of the estrogen receptor. *Cold Spring Harb Symp Quant Biol* 1986; 51 Pt 2:751-8.

[30] Kuiper GG, Enmark E, Pelto-Huikko M, Nilsson S, Gustafsson JA. Cloning of a novel receptor expressed in rat prostate and ovary. *Proc Natl Acad Sci U S A* 1996; 93:5925-30.

[31] Kuiper GG, Carlsson B, Grandien K, *et al.* Comparison of the ligand binding specificity and transcript tissue distribution of estrogen receptors alpha and beta. *Endocrinology* 1997; 138:863-70.

[32] Roy JR, Chakraborty S, Chakraborty TR. Estrogen-like endocrine disrupting chemicals affecting puberty in humans--a review. *Med Sci Monit* 2009; 15:RA137-45.

[33] Faulds MH, Zhao C, Dahlman-Wright K, Gustafsson JA. The diversity of sex steroid action: regulation of metabolism by estrogen signaling. *Journal of Endocrinology* 2012; 212:3-12.

[34] Zhao C, Dahlman-Wright K, Gustafsson JA. Estrogen receptor beta: an overview and update. *Nucl Recept Signal* 2008; 6:e003.

[35] Nilsson S, Makela S, Treuter E, *et al.* Mechanisms of estrogen action. *Physiol Rev* 2001; 81:1535-65.

[36] Metivier R, Reid G, Gannon F. Transcription in four dimensions: nuclear receptor-directed initiation of gene expression. *EMBO Rep* 2006; 7:161-7.

[37] Gruber CJ, Gruber DM, Gruber IM, Wieser F, Huber JC. Anatomy of the estrogen response element. *Trends Endocrinol Metab* 2004; 15:73-8.

[38] Aranda A, Pascual A. Nuclear hormone receptors and gene expression. *Physiol Rev* 2001; 81:1269-304.

[39] Foryst-Ludwig A, Kintscher U. Metabolic impact of estrogen signalling through ERalpha and ERbeta. *J Steroid Biochem Mol Biol* 2010; 122:74-81.

[40] Lubahn DB, Moyer JS, Golding TS, Couse JF, Korach KS, Smithies O. Alteration of reproductive function but not prenatal sexual development after insertional disruption of the mouse estrogen receptor gene. *Proc Natl Acad Sci U S A* 1993; 90:11162-6.

[41] Fisher CR, Graves KH, Parlow AF, Simpson ER. Characterization of mice deficient in aromatase (ArKO) because of targeted disruption of the cyp19 gene. *Proc Natl Acad Sci U S A* 1998; 95:6965-70.

[42] Krege JH, Hodgin JB, Couse JF, *et al.* Generation and reproductive phenotypes of mice lacking estrogen receptor beta. *Proc Natl Acad Sci U S A* 1998; 95:15677-82.

[43] Couse JF, Korach KS. Reproductive phenotypes in the estrogen receptor-alpha knockout mouse. *Ann Endocrinol (Paris)* 1999; 60:143-8.

[44] Smith EP, Boyd J, Frank GR, *et al.* Estrogen resistance caused by a mutation in the estrogen-receptor gene in a man. *N Engl J Med* 1994; 331:1056-61.

[45] Grumbach MM, Auchus RJ. Estrogen: consequences and implications of human mutations in synthesis and action. *J Clin Endocrinol Metab* 1999; 84:4677-94.

[46] Revankar CM, Cimino DF, Sklar LA, Arterburn JB, Prossnitz ER. A transmembrane intracellular estrogen receptor mediates rapid cell signaling. *Science* 2005; 307:1625-30.

[47] Filardo E, Quinn J, Pang Y, *et al.* Activation of the novel estrogen receptor G protein-coupled receptor 30 (GPR30) at the plasma membrane. *Endocrinology* 2007; 148:3236-45.

[48] Carmeci C, Thompson DA, Ring HZ, Francke U, Weigel RJ. Identification of a gene (GPR30) with homology to the G-protein-coupled receptor superfamily associated with estrogen receptor expression in breast cancer. *Genomics* 1997; 45:607-17.

[49] Filardo EJ, Quinn JA, Bland KI, Frackelton AR, Jr. Estrogen-induced activation of Erk-1 and Erk-2 requires the G protein-coupled receptor homolog, GPR30, and occurs via trans-activation of the epidermal growth factor receptor through release of HB-EGF. *Mol Endocrinol* 2000; 14:1649-60.

[50] Chen Z, Yuhanna IS, Galcheva-Gargova Z, Karas RH, Mendelsohn ME, Shaul PW. Estrogen receptor alpha mediates the nongenomic activation of endothelial nitric oxide synthase by estrogen. *Journal of Clinical Investigation* 1999; 103:401-6.

[51] Levin ER. Cellular Functions of the Plasma Membrane Estrogen Receptor. *Trends Endocrinol Metab* 1999; 10:374-7.

[52] Norfleet AM, Thomas ML, Gametchu B, Watson CS. Estrogen receptor-alpha detected on the plasma membrane of aldehyde-fixed GH3/B6/F10 rat pituitary tumor cells by enzyme-linked immuno-cytochemistry. *Endocrinology* 1999; 140:3805-14.

[53] Aronica SM, Kraus WL, Katzenellenbogen BS. Estrogen action via the cAMP signaling pathway: stimulation of adenylate cyclase and cAMP-regulated gene transcription. *Proc Natl Acad Sci U S A* 1994; 91:8517-21.

[54] Doolan CM, Harvey BJ. A Galphas protein-coupled membrane receptor, distinct from the classical oestrogen receptor, transduces rapid effects of oestradiol on [Ca2+]i in female rat distal colon. *Mol Cell Endocrinol* 2003; 199:87-103.

[55] Carlezon WA, Jr., Duman RS, Nestler EJ. The many faces of CREB. *Trends Neurosci* 2005; 28:436-45.

[56] Anwar A, McTernan PG, Anderson LA, *et al.* Site-specific regulation of oestrogen receptor-alpha and -beta by oestradiol in human adipose tissue. *Diabetes Obesity & Metabolism* 2001; 3:338-49.

[57] Dos Santos EG, Dieudonne MN, Pecquery R, Le Moal V, Giudicelli Y, Lacasa D. Rapid nongenomic E2 effects on p42/p44 MAPK, activator protein-1, and cAMP response element binding protein in rat white adipocytes. *Endocrinology* 2002; 143:930-40.

[58] Dieudonne MN, Leneveu MC, Giudicelli Y, Pecquery R. Evidence for functional estrogen receptors alpha and beta in human adipose cells: regional specificities and regulation by estrogens. *Am J Physiol Cell Physiol* 2004; 286:C655-61.

[59] Cooke PS, Heine PA, Taylor JA, Lubahn DB. The role of estrogen and estrogen receptor-alpha in male adipose tissue. *Molecular and Cellular Endocrinology* 2001; 178:147-54.

[60] Giguere V. Transcriptional control of energy homeostasis by the estrogen-related receptors. *Endocrine Reviews* 2008; 29:677-96.

[61] Fu M, Sun T, Bookout AL, *et al.* A Nuclear Receptor Atlas: 3T3-L1 adipogenesis. *Mol Endocrinol* 2005; 19:2437-50.

[62] Barish GD, Downes M, Alaynick WA, *et al.* A Nuclear Receptor Atlas: macrophage activation. *Mol Endocrinol* 2005; 19:2466-77.

[63] Frasor J, Barnett DH, Danes JM, Hess R, Parlow AF, Katzenellenbogen BS. Response-specific and ligand dose-dependent modulation of estrogen receptor (ER) alpha activity by ERbeta in the uterus. *Endocrinology* 2003; 144:3159-66.

[64] Meseguer A, Puche C, Cabero A. Sex steroid biosynthesis in white adipose tissue. *Hormone and Metabolic Research* 2002; 34:731-6.

[65] Belanger C, Luu-The V, Dupont P, Tchernof A. Adipose tissue intracrinology: potential importance of local androgen/estrogen metabolism in the regulation of adiposity. *Hormone and Metabolic Research* 2002; 34:737-45.

[66] Jones MEE, McInnes KJ, Boon WC, Simpson ER. Estrogen and adiposity - Utilizing models of aromatase deficiency to explore the relationship. *Journal of Steroid Biochemistry and Molecular Biology* 2007; 106:3-7.

[67] Jones MEE, Boon WC, Proietto J, Simpson ER. Of mice and men: the evolving phenotype of aromatase deficiency. *Trends in Endocrinology and Metabolism* 2006; 17:53-62.

[68] Carani C, Qin K, Simoni M, *et al.* Effect of testosterone and estradiol in a man with aromatase deficiency. *New England Journal of Medicine* 1997; 337:91-5.

[69] Alberti KG, Eckel RH, Grundy SM, *et al.* Harmonizing the metabolic syndrome: a joint interim statement of the International Diabetes Federation Task Force on Epidemiology and Prevention; National Heart, Lung, and Blood Institute; American Heart Association; World Heart Federation; International Atherosclerosis Society; and International Association for the Study of Obesity. *Circulation* 2009; 120:1640-5.

[70] Sato K, Matsuki N, Ohno Y, Nakazawa K. Estrogens inhibit l-glutamate uptake activity of astrocytes via membrane estrogen receptor alpha. *J Neurochem* 2003; 86:1498-505.

[71] Heine PA, Taylor JA, Iwamoto GA, Lubahn DB, Cooke PS. Increased adipose tissue in male and female estrogen receptor-alpha knockout mice. *Proceedings of the National Academy of Sciences of the United States of America* 2000; 97:12729-34.

[72] Danilovich N, Babu PS, Xing W, Gerdes M, Krishnamurthy H, Sairam MR. Estrogen deficiency, obesity, and skeletal abnormalities in follicle-stimulating hormone receptor knockout (FORKO) female mice. *Endocrinology* 2000; 141:4295-308.

[73] Naaz A, Zakroczymski M, Heine P, *et al.* Effect of ovariectomy on adipose tissue of mice in the absence of estrogen receptor alpha (ERalpha): a potential role for estrogen receptor beta (ERbeta). *Hormone and Metabolic Research* 2002; 34:758-63.

[74] Foryst-Ludwig A, Clemenz M, Hohmann S, *et al.* Metabolic Actions of Estrogen Receptor Beta (ER beta) are Mediated by a Negative Cross-Talk with PPAR gamma. *Plos Genetics* 2008; 4.

[75] Nilsson S, Gustafsson JA. Estrogen receptors: therapies targeted to receptor subtypes. *Clin Pharmacol Ther*; 89:44-55.

[76]   Haas E, Bhattacharya I, Brailoiu E, *et al.* Regulatory role of G protein-coupled estrogen receptor for vascular function and obesity. *Circ Res* 2009; 104:288-91.

[77]   Wang C, Dehghani B, Magrisso IJ, *et al.* GPR30 contributes to estrogen-induced thymic atrophy. *Mol Endocrinol* 2008; 22:636-48.

[78]   Hugo ER, Brandebourg TD, Woo JG, Loftus J, Alexander JW, Ben-Jonathan N. Bisphenol A at environmentally relevant doses inhibits adiponectin release from human adipose tissue explants and adipocytes. *Environ Health Perspect* 2008; 116:1642-7.

[79]   Murase Y, Kobayashi J, Nohara A, *et al.* Raloxifene promotes adipocyte differentiation of 3T3-L1 cells. *Eur J Pharmacol* 2006; 538:1-4.

[80]   Martensson UEA, Salehi SA, Windahl S, *et al.* Deletion of the G Protein-Coupled Receptor 30 Impairs Glucose Tolerance, Reduces Bone Growth, Increases Blood Pressure, and Eliminates Estradiol-Stimulated Insulin Release in Female Mice. *Endocrinology* 2009; 150:687-98.

[81]   Stubbins RE, Holcomb VB, Hong J, Nunez NP. Estrogen modulates abdominal adiposity and protects female mice from obesity and impaired glucose tolerance. *Eur J Nutr* 2011.

[82]   Riant E, Waget A, Cogo H, Arnal JF, Burcelin R, Gourdy P. Estrogens protect against high-fat diet-induced insulin resistance and glucose intolerance in mice. *Endocrinology* 2009; 150:2109-17.

[83]   Sudhir K, Chou TM, Chatterjee K, *et al.* Premature coronary artery disease associated with a disruptive mutation in the estrogen receptor gene in a man. *Circulation* 1997; 96:3774-7.

[84]   Schuit SC, Oei HH, Witteman JC, *et al.* Estrogen receptor alpha gene polymorphisms and risk of myocardial infarction. *JAMA* 2004; 291:2969-77.

[85]   Yoshihara R, Utsunomiya K, Gojo A, *et al.* Association of polymorphism of estrogen receptor-alpha gene with circulating levels of adiponectin in postmenopausal women with type 2 diabetes. *J Atheroscler Thromb* 2009; 16:250-5.

[86]   Lamon-Fava S, Asztalos BF, Howard TD, *et al.* Association of polymorphisms in genes involved in lipoprotein metabolism with plasma concentrations of remnant lipoproteins and HDL subpopulations before and after hormone therapy in postmenopausal women. *Clin Endocrinol (Oxf)*; 72:169-75.

[87]   Eastwood H, Brown KM, Markovic D, Pieri LF. Variation in the ESR1 and ESR2 genes and genetic susceptibility to anorexia nervosa. *Mol Psychiatry* 2002; 7:86-9.

[88] Nilsson S, Koehler KF, Gustafsson JA. Development of subtype-selective oestrogen receptor-based therapeutics. *Nat Rev Drug Discov* 2011; 10:778-92.

[89] Mansur Ade P, Nogueira CC, Strunz CM, Aldrighi JM, Ramires JA. Genetic polymorphisms of estrogen receptors in patients with premature coronary artery disease. *Arch Med Res* 2005; 36:511-7.

[90] Regitz-Zagrosek V, Lehmkuhl E, Weickert MO. Gender differences in the metabolic syndrome and their role for cardiovascular disease. *Clinical Research in Cardiology* 2006; 95:136-47.

[91] Stork S, van der Schouw YT, Grobbee DE, Bots ML. Estrogen, inflammation and cardiovascular risk in women: a critical appraisal. *Trends in Endocrinology and Metabolism* 2004; 15:66-72.

[92] Lobo RA. Inflammation, coronary artery disease, and hormones. *Menopause* 2008; 15:1036-8.

[93] Cignarella A, Kratz M, Bolego C. Emerging role of estrogen in the control of cardiometabolic disease. *Trends Pharmacol Sci*; 31:183-9.

[94] Salama SA, Kamel MW, Diaz-Arrastia CR, *et al.* Effect of tumor necrosis factor-alpha on estrogen metabolism and endometrial cells: potential physiological and pathological relevance. *J Clin Endocrinol Metab* 2009; 94:285-93.

[95] Roncari DA. Metabolism of estrogens in rat adipose tissue. *Endocrinology* 1967; 80:1160-3.

[96] Anderson LA, McTernan PG, Barnett AH, Kumar S. The effects of androgens and estrogens on preadipocyte proliferation in human adipose tissue: Influence of gender and site. *Journal of Clinical Endocrinology & Metabolism* 2001; 86:5045-51.

[97] Heine PA, Lubahn DB, Keisler DH, Hufford M, Cooke PS. Role of estrogen receptor alpha (ER alpha) in white adipose tissue (WAT) deposition in mice. *Biology of Reproduction* 2000; 62:306-7.

[98] Jones ME, Thorburn AW, Britt KL, *et al.* Aromatase-deficient (ArKO) mice have a phenotype of increased adiposity. *Proc Natl Acad Sci U S A* 2000; 97:12735-40.

[99] Bouchard C, Despres JP, Mauriege P. Genetic and nongenetic determinants of regional fat distribution. *Endocrine Reviews* 1993; 14:72-93.

[100] Meinhardt UJ, Ho KK. Modulation of growth hormone action by sex steroids. *Clin Endocrinol (Oxf)* 2006; 65:413-22.

[101] Horlick MB, Rosenbaum M, Nicolson M, *et al.* Effect of puberty on the relationship between circulating leptin and body composition. *J Clin Endocrinol Metab* 2000; 85:2509-18.

[102] Nindl BC, Scoville CR, Sheehan KM, Leone CD, Mello RP. Gender differences in regional body composition and somatotrophic influences of IGF-I and leptin. *J Appl Physiol* 2002; 92:1611-8.

[103] Sieminska L, Wojciechowska C, Niedziolka D, *et al.* Effect of postmenopause and hormone replacement therapy on serum adiponectin levels. *Metabolism* 2005; 54:1610-4.

[104] Andersen KK, Frystyk J, Wolthers OD, Heuck C, Flyvbjerg A. Gender differences of oligomers and total adiponectin during puberty: A cross-sectional study of 859 Danish school children. *Journal of Clinical Endocrinology & Metabolism* 2007; 92:1857-62.

[105] Asai K, Hiki N, Mimura Y, Ogawa T, Unou K, Kaminishi M. Gender differences in cytokine secretion by human peripheral blood mononuclear cells: role of estrogen in modulating LPS-induced cytokine secretion in an ex vivo septic model. *Shock* 2001; 16:340-3.

[106] Garaulet M, Hernandez-Morante JJ, Tebar FJ, Zamora S. Anthropometric indexes for visceral fat estimation in overweight/obese women attending to age and menopausal status. *J Physiol Biochem* 2006; 62:245-52.

[107] Haffner SM, Katz MS, Dunn JF. Increased upper body and overall adiposity is associated with decreased sex hormone binding globulin in postmenopausal women. *Int J Obes* 1991; 15:471-8.

[108] Hautanen A. Synthesis and regulation of sex hormone-binding globulin in obesity. *Int J Obes Relat Metab Disord* 2000; 24 Suppl 2:S64-70.

[109] De Pergola G, Zamboni M, Sciaraffia M, *et al.* Body fat accumulation is possibly responsible for lower dehydroepiandrosterone circulating levels in premenopausal obese women. *Int J Obes Relat Metab Disord* 1996; 20:1105-10.

[110] Hernandez-Morante JJ, Perez-de-Heredia F, Lujan JA, Zamora S, Garaulet M. Role of DHEA-S on body fat distribution: gender- and depot-specific stimulation of adipose tissue lipolysis. *Steroids* 2008; 73:209-15.

[111] Kant AK, Graubard BI. Secular trends in patterns of self-reported food consumption of adult Americans: NHANES 1971-1975 to NHANES 1999-2002. *Am J Clin Nutr* 2006; 84:1215-23.

[112] Davidsen L, Vistisen B, Astrup A. Impact of the menstrual cycle on determinants of energy balance: a putative role in weight loss attempts. *Int J Obes (Lond)* 2007; 31:1777-85.

[113] Asarian L, Geary N. Modulation of appetite by gonadal steroid hormones. *Philos Trans R Soc Lond B Biol Sci* 2006; 361:1251-63.

[114] Geary N, Asarian L, Korach KS, Pfaff DW, Ogawa S. Deficits in E2-dependent control of feeding, weight gain, and cholecystokinin satiation in ER-alpha null mice. *Endocrinology* 2001; 142:4751-7.

[115] Schneider JE. Energy balance and reproduction. *Physiol Behav* 2004; 81:289-317.

[116] Shen L, Wang DQ, Lo CM, *et al.* Estradiol increases the anorectic effect of central apolipoprotein A-IV. *Endocrinology*; 151:3163-8.

[117] Roepke TA. Oestrogen Modulates Hypothalamic Control of Energy Homeostasis Through Multiple Mechanisms. *Journal of Neuro-endocrinology* 2009; 21:141-50.

[118] Musatov S, Chen W, Pfaff DW, *et al.* Silencing of estrogen receptor alpha in the ventromedial nucleus of hypothalamus leads to metabolic syndrome. *Proc Natl Acad Sci U S A* 2007; 104:2501-6.

[119] Liang YQ, Akishita M, Kim S, *et al.* Estrogen receptor beta is involved in the anorectic action of estrogen. *International Journal of Obesity* 2002; 26:1103-9.

[120] Chumlea WC, Knittle JL, Roche AF, Siervogel RM, Webb P. Size and number of adipocytes and measures of body fat in boys and girls 10 to 18 years of age. *Am J Clin Nutr* 1981; 34:1791-7.

[121] Sjostrom L, Smith U, Krotkiewski M, Bjorntorp P. Cellularity in different regions of adipose tissue in young men and women. *Metabolism-Clinical and Experimental* 1972; 21:1143-53.

[122] O'Sullivan AJ. Does oestrogen allow women to store fat more efficiently? A biological advantage for fertility and gestation. *Obesity Reviews* 2009; 10:168-77.

[123] Hamosh M, Hamosh P. The effect of estrogen on the lipoprotein lipase activity of rat adipose tissue. *Journal of Clinical Investigation* 1975; 55:1132-5.

[124] Palin SL, McTernan PG, Anderson LA, Sturdee DW, Barnett AH, Kumar S. 17Beta-estradiol and anti-estrogen ICI:compound 182,780 regulate expression of lipoprotein lipase and hormone-sensitive lipase in isolated subcutaneous abdominal adipocytes. *Metabolism* 2003; 52:383-8.

[125] Ackerman GE, MacDonald PC, Gudelsky G, Mendelson CR, Simpson ER. Potentiation of epinephrine-induced lipolysis by catechol estrogens and their methoxy derivatives. *Endocrinology* 1981; 109:2084-8.

[126] Misso ML, Murata Y, Boon WC, Jones MEE, Britt KL, Simpson ER. Cellular and molecular characterization of the adipose phenotype of the aromatase-deficient mouse. *Endocrinology* 2003; 144:1474-80.

[127] Vegeto E, Bonincontro C, Pollio G, *et al.* Estrogen prevents the lipopolysaccharide-induced inflammatory response in microglia. *J Neurosci* 2001; 21:1809-18.

[128] Pozzi S, Benedusi V, Maggi A, Vegeto E. Estrogen action in neuro-protection and brain inflammation. *Estrogens and Human Diseases* 2006; 1089:302-23.

[129] Turgeon JL, Carr MC, Maki PM, Mendelsohn ME, Wise PM. Complex actions of sex steroids in adipose tissue, the cardiovascular system, and brain: Insights from basic science and clinical studies. *Endocrine Reviews* 2006; 27:575-605.

[130] Stein B, Yang MX. Repression of the Interleukin-6 Promoter by Estrogen-Receptor Is Mediated by Nf-Kappa-B and C/Ebp-Beta. *Mol Cell Biol* 1995; 15:4971-9.

[131] Ghisletti S, Meda C, Maggi A, Vegeto E. 17beta-estradiol inhibits inflammatory gene expression by controlling NF-kappaB intracellular localization. *Mol Cell Biol* 2005; 25:2957-68.

[132] Murphy AJ, Guyre PM, Wira CR, Pioli PA. Estradiol regulates expression of estrogen receptor ERalpha46 in human macrophages. *PLoS One* 2009; 4:e5539.

[133] Blasko E, Haskell CA, Leung S, *et al.* Beneficial role of the GPR30 agonist G-1 in an animal model of multiple sclerosis. *J Neuroimmunol* 2009; 214:67-77.

[134] Deshpande R, Khalili H, Pergolizzi RG, Michael SD, Chang MD. Estradiol down-regulates LPS-induced cytokine production and NFkB activation in murine macrophages. *Am J Reprod Immunol* 1997; 38:46-54.

[135] Frazier-Jessen MR, Kovacs EJ. Estrogen modulation of JE/monocyte chemoattractant protein-1 mRNA expression in murine macrophages. *J Immunol* 1995; 154:1838-45.

[136] Dantas AP, Sandberg K. Estrogen regulation of tumor necrosis factor-alpha: a missing link between menopause and cardiovascular risk in women? *Hypertension* 2005; 46:21-2.

[137] Arenas IA, Armstrong SJ, Xu Y, Davidge ST. Chronic tumor necrosis factor-alpha inhibition enhances NO modulation of vascular function in estrogen-deficient rats. *Hypertension* 2005; 46:76-81.

[138] Geer EB, Shen W. Gender Differences in Insulin Resistance, Body Composition, and Energy Balance. *Gender Medicine* 2009; 6:60-75.

[139] Szalowska E, Dijkstra M, Elferink MG, *et al.* Comparative analysis of the human hepatic and adipose tissue transcriptomes during LPS-induced inflammation leads to the identification of differential biological pathways and candidate biomarkers. *BMC Med Genomics*; 4:71.

[140] Koh KK, Ahn JY, Kang MH, *et al.* Effects of hormone replacement therapy on plaque stability, inflammation, and fibrinolysis in hypertensive or overweight postmenopausal women. *Am J Cardiol* 2001; 88:1423-6, A8.

[141] Rogers A, Eastell R. The effect of 17beta-estradiol on production of cytokines in cultures of peripheral blood. *Bone* 2001; 29:30-4.

[142] Newbold RR, Padilla-Banks E, Jefferson WN, Heindel JJ. Effects of endocrine disruptors on obesity. *Int J Androl* 2008; 31:201-8.

[143] Baillie-Hamilton PF. Chemical toxins: a hypothesis to explain the global obesity epidemic. *J Altern Complement Med* 2002; 8:185-92.

[144] Bougneres P. Genetics of obesity and type 2 diabetes: tracking pathogenic traits during the predisease period. *Diabetes* 2002; 51 Suppl 3:S295-303.

[145] Heindel JJ. Endocrine disruptors and the obesity epidemic. *Toxicol Sci* 2003; 76:247-9.

[146] Grun F, Blumberg B. Environmental obesogens: organotins and endocrine disruption via nuclear receptor signaling. *Endocrinology* 2006; 147:S50-5.

[147] Grun F, Watanabe H, Zamanian Z, *et al.* Endocrine-disrupting organotin compounds are potent inducers of adipogenesis in vertebrates. *Mol Endocrinol* 2006; 20:2141-55.

[148] Grun F, Blumberg B. Perturbed nuclear receptor signaling by environmental obesogens as emerging factors in the obesity crisis. *Rev Endocr Metab Disord* 2007; 8:161-71.

[149] Carson R. *Silent Spring.* 1962; Houghton Mifflin United States.

[150] Kojima H, Sata F, Takeuchi S, Sueyoshi T, Nagai T. Comparative study of human and mouse pregnane X receptor agonistic activity in 200 pesticides using in vitro reporter gene assays. *Toxicology*; 280:77-87.

[151] Gutendorf B, Westendorf J. Comparison of an array of in vitro assays for the assessment of the estrogenic potential of natural and synthetic estrogens, phytoestrogens and xenoestrogens. *Toxicology* 2001; 166:79-89.

[152] Witorsch RJ. Low-dose in utero effects of xenoestrogens in mice and their relevance to humans: an analytical review of the literature. *Food Chem Toxicol* 2002; 40:905-12.

[153] Swedenborg E, Ruegg J, Makela S, Pongratz I. Endocrine disruptive chemicals: mechanisms of action and involvement in metabolic disorders. *J Mol Endocrinol* 2009; 43:1-10.

[154] Brzozowski AM, Pike AC, Dauter Z, *et al.* Molecular basis of agonism and antagonism in the oestrogen receptor. *Nature* 1997; 389:753-8.

[155] Blair RM, Fang H, Branham WS, *et al.* The estrogen receptor relative binding affinities of 188 natural and xenochemicals: structural diversity of ligands. *Toxicol Sci* 2000; 54:138-53.

[156] Adeoya-Osiguwa SA, Markoulaki S, Pocock V, Milligan SR, Fraser LR. 17beta-Estradiol and environmental estrogens significantly affect mammalian sperm function. *Human Reproduction* 2003; 18:100-7.

[157] Nadal A, Ropero AB, Laribi O, Maillet M, Fuentes E, Soria B. Nongenomic actions of estrogens and xenoestrogens by binding at a plasma membrane receptor unrelated to estrogen receptor alpha and estrogen receptor beta. *Proc Natl Acad Sci U S A* 2000; 97:11603-8.

[158] Ruehlmann DO, Steinert JR, Valverde MA, Jacob R, Mann GE. Environmental estrogenic pollutants induce acute vascular relaxation by inhibiting L-type Ca2+ channels in smooth muscle cells. *FASEB J* 1998; 12:613-9.

[159] Watson CS, Campbell CH, Gametchu B. Membrane oestrogen receptors on rat pituitary tumour cells: immuno-identification and responses to oestradiol and xenoestrogens. *Exp Physiol* 1999; 84:1013-22.

[160] Wober J, Weisswange I, Vollmer G. Stimulation of alkaline phosphatase activity in Ishikawa cells induced by various phytoestrogens and synthetic estrogens. *J Steroid Biochem Mol Biol* 2002; 83:227-33.

[161] Watson CS, Pappas TC, Gametchu B. The other estrogen receptor in the plasma membrane: implications for the actions of environmental estrogens. *Environ Health Perspect* 1995; 103 Suppl 7:41-50.

[162] Bulayeva NN, Watson CS. Xenoestrogen-induced ERK-1 and ERK-2 activation via multiple membrane-initiated signaling pathways. *Environ Health Perspect* 2004; 112:1481-7.

[163] Bulayeva NN, Gametchu B, Watson CS. Quantitative measurement of estrogen-induced ERK 1 and 2 activation via multiple membrane-initiated signaling pathways. *Steroids* 2004; 69:181-92.

[164] Thomas P, Pang Y, Filardo EJ, Dong J. Identity of an estrogen membrane receptor coupled to a G protein in human breast cancer cells. *Endocrinology* 2005; 146:624-32.

[165] Quesada I, Fuentes E, Viso-Leon MC, Soria B, Ripoll C, Nadal A. Low doses of the endocrine disruptor bisphenol-A and the native hormone 17beta-estradiol rapidly activate transcription factor CREB. *FASEB J* 2002; 16:1671-3.

[166] Canesi L, Lorusso LC, Ciacci C, Betti M, Zampini M, Gallo G. Environmental estrogens can affect the function of mussel hemocytes through rapid modulation of kinase pathways. *Gen Comp Endocrinol* 2004; 138:58-69.

[167] Elobeid MA, Allison DB. Putative environmental-endocrine disruptors and obesity: a review. *Curr Opin Endocrinol Diabetes Obes* 2008; 15:403-8.

[168] Oseni T, Patel R, Pyle J, Jordan VC. Selective estrogen receptor modulators and phytoestrogens. *Planta Med* 2008; 74:1656-65.

[169] Newbold RR. Impact of environmental endocrine disrupting chemicals on the development of obesity. *Hormones (Athens)* 2010; 9:206-17.

[170] Blake C, Fabick KM, Setchell KD, Lund TD, Lephart ED. Neuromodulation by soy diets or equol: anti-depressive & anti-obesity-like influences, age- & hormone-dependent effects. *BMC Neurosci*; 12:28.

[171] Penza M, Montani C, Romani A, *et al.* Genistein affects adipose tissue deposition in a dose-dependent and gender-specific manner. *Endocrinology* 2006; 147:5740-51.

[172] Park HJ, Della-Fera MA, Hausman DB, Rayalam S, Ambati S, Baile CA. Genistein inhibits differentiation of primary human adipocytes. *J Nutr Biochem* 2009; 20:140-8.

[173] Heim M, Frank O, Kampmann G, *et al.* The phytoestrogen genistein enhances osteogenesis and represses adipogenic differentiation of human primary bone marrow stromal cells. *Endocrinology* 2004; 145:848-59.

[174] Szkudelska K, Nogowski L, Szkudelski T. Genistein affects lipogenesis and lipolysis in isolated rat adipocytes. *J Steroid Biochem Mol Biol* 2000; 75:265-71.

[175] Harmon AW, Harp JB. Differential effects of flavonoids on 3T3-L1 adipogenesis and lipolysis. *Am J Physiol Cell Physiol* 2001; 280:C807-13.

[176] Rogers NH, Perfield JW, 2nd, Strissel KJ, Obin MS, Greenberg AS. Reduced energy expenditure and increased inflammation are early events in the development of ovariectomy-induced obesity. *Endocrinology* 2009; 150:2161-8.

[177] Wade GN, Gray JM, Bartness TJ. Gonadal Influences on Adiposity. *International Journal of Obesity* 1985; 9:83-92.

[178] Lephart ED, Porter JP, Lund TD, *et al.* Dietary isoflavones alter regulatory behaviors, metabolic hormones and neuroendocrine function in Long-Evans male rats. *Nutr Metab (Lond)* 2004; 1:16.

[179] Kim HK, Nelson-Dooley C, Della-Fera MA, *et al.* Genistein decreases food intake, body weight, and fat pad weight and causes adipose tissue apoptosis in ovariectomized female mice. *J Nutr* 2006; 136:409-14.

[180] Naaz A, Yellayi S, Zakroczymski MA, *et al.* The soy isoflavone genistein decreases adipose deposition in mice. *Endocrinology* 2003; 144:3315-20.

[181] Limer JL, Speirs V. Phyto-oestrogens and breast cancer chemoprevention. *Breast Cancer Res* 2004; 6:119-27.

[182] Dang ZC, Papapoulos S, Lowik C. Phytoestrogens enhance osteogenesis and concurrently inhibit adipogenesis. *Journal of Nutrition* 2002; 132:617s-s.

[183] Thomas P, Dong J. Binding and activation of the seven-transmembrane estrogen receptor GPR30 by environmental estrogens: a potential novel mechanism of endocrine disruption. *J Steroid Biochem Mol Biol* 2006; 102:175-9.

[184] Maggiolini M, Picard D. The unfolding stories of GPR30, a new membrane-bound estrogen receptor. *Journal of Endocrinology* 2010; 204:105-14.

[185] Wittassek M, Wiesmuller GA, Koch HM, *et al.* Internal phthalate exposure over the last two decades - A retrospective human biomonitoring study. *International Journal of Hygiene and Environmental Health* 2007; 210:319-33.

[186] Calafat AM, Kuklenyik Z, Reidy JA, Caudill SP, Ekong J, Needham LL. Urinary concentrations of bisphenol A and 4-nonylphenol in a human reference population. *Environmental Health Perspectives* 2005; 113:391-5.

[187] Pelletier C, Doucet E, Imbeault P, Tremblay A. Associations between weight loss-induced changes in plasma organochlorine concentrations, serum T-3 concentration, and resting metabolic rate. *Toxicological Sciences* 2002; 67:46-51.

[188] Chevrier J, Dewailly E, Ayotte P, Mauriege P, Despres JP, Tremblay A. Body weight loss increases plasma and adipose tissue concentrations of potentially toxic pollutants in obese individuals. *International Journal of Obesity* 2000; 24:1272-8.

[189] Goncharov A, Haase RF, Santiago-Rivera A, *et al.* High serum PCBs are associated with elevation of serum lipids and cardiovascular disease in a Native American population. *Environmental Research* 2008; 106:226-39.

[190] Pelletier C, Despres JP, Tremblay A. Plasma organochlorine concentrations in endurance athletes and obese individuals. *Medicine and Science in Sports and Exercise* 2002; 34:1971-5.

[191] Takeuchi T, Tsutsumi O, Ikezuki Y, Takai Y, Taketani Y. Positive relationship between androgen and the endocrine disruptor, bisphenol A, in normal women and women with ovarian dysfunction. *Endocrine Journal* 2004; 51:165-9.

[192] Lee DH, Lee IK, Song K, *et al.* A strong dose-response relation between serum concentrations of persistent organic pollutants and diabetes: results from the National Health and Examination Survey 1999-2002. *Diabetes Care* 2006; 29:1638-44.

[193] Lee DH, Lee IK, Porta M, Steffes M, Jacobs DR, Jr. Relationship between serum concentrations of persistent organic pollutants and the prevalence of metabolic syndrome among non-diabetic adults: results from the National Health and Nutrition Examination Survey 1999-2002. *Diabetologia* 2007; 50:1841-51.

[194] Lee MJ, Lin H, Liu CW, *et al.* Octylphenol stimulates resistin gene expression in 3T3-L1 adipocytes via the estrogen receptor and extracellular signal-regulated kinase pathways. *Am J Physiol Cell Physiol* 2008; 294:C1542-51.

[195] Vandenberg LN, Hauser R, Marcus M, Olea N, Welshons WV. Human exposure to bisphenol A (BPA). *Reproductive Toxicology* 2007; 24:139-77.

[196] Shin BS, Kim CH, Jun YS, *et al.* Physiologically based pharmacokinetics of bisphenol A. *J Toxicol Environ Health A* 2004; 67:1971-85.

[197] Nunez AA, Kannan K, Giesy JP, Fang J, Clemens LG. Effects of bisphenol A on energy balance and accumulation in brown adipose tissue in rats. *Chemosphere* 2001; 42:917-22.

[198] Seidlova-Wuttke D, Jarry H, Christoffel J, Rimoldi G, Wuttke W. Effects of bisphenol-A (BPA), dibutylphtalate (DBP), benzophenone-2 (BP2), procymidone (Proc), and linurone (Lin) on fat tissue, a variety of hormones and metabolic parameters: A 3 months comparison with effects of estradiol (E2) in ovariectomized (ovx) rats. *Toxicology* 2005; 213:13-24.

[199] Masuno H, Kidani T, Sekiya K, *et al.* Bisphenol A in combination with insulin can accelerate the conversion of 3T3-L1 fibroblasts to adipocytes. *J Lipid Res* 2002; 43:676-84.

[200] Sakurai K, Kawazuma M, Adachi T, *et al.* Bisphenol A affects glucose transport in mouse 3T3-F442A adipocytes. *Br J Pharmacol* 2004; 141:209-14.

[201] Gesta S, Tseng YH, Kahn CR. Developmental origin of fat: tracking obesity to its source. *Cell* 2007; 131:242-56.

[202] Newbold RR, Padilla-Banks E, Snyder RJ, Phillips TM, Jefferson WN. Developmental exposure to endocrine disruptors and the obesity epidemic. *Reprod Toxicol* 2007; 23:290-6.

[203] Zimmerman SA, Clevenger WR, Brimhall BB, Bradshaw WS. Diethylstilbestrol-induced perinatal lethality in the rat. II. Perturbation of parturition. *Biology of Reproduction* 1991; 44:583-9.

[204] Clevenger WR, Cornwall GA, Carter MW, Bradshaw WS. Diethylstilbestrol-induced perinatal lethality in the rat. I. Relationship to reduced maternal weight gain. *Biology of Reproduction* 1991; 44:575-82.

[205] Ema M, Miyawaki E. Effects on development of the reproductive system in male offspring of rats given butyl benzyl phthalate during late pregnancy. *Reprod Toxicol* 2002; 16:71-6.

[206] Rubin BS, Murray MK, Damassa DA, King JC, Soto AM. Perinatal exposure to low doses of bisphenol A affects body weight, patterns of estrous cyclicity, and plasma LH levels. *Environ Health Perspect* 2001; 109:675-80.

[207] Givens ML, Small CM, Terrell ML, *et al.* Maternal exposure to poly-brominated and polychlorinated biphenyls: Infant birth weight and gestational age. *Chemosphere* 2007; 69:1295-304.

[208] Fein GG, Jacobson JL, Jacobson SW, Schwartz PM, Dowler JK. Prenatal Exposure to Polychlorinated-Biphenyls - Effects on Birth Size and Gestational-Age. *Journal of Pediatrics* 1984; 105:315-20.

[209] Baker DJ, Fuhrman J, Renter F. Perspectives on organizational growth. *Ment Retard* 2002; 40:477-80.

[210] Hochberg Z, Feil R, Constancia M, *et al.* Child health, developmental plasticity, and epigenetic programming. *Endocrine Reviews* 2002; 32:159-224.

[211] Bromer JG, Wu J, Zhou Y, Taylor HS. Hypermethylation of homeobox A10 by in utero diethylstilbestrol exposure: an epigenetic mechanism for altered developmental programming. *Endocrinology* 2009; 150:3376-82.

[212] Newbold RR. Lessons learned from perinatal exposure to diethylstilbestrol. *Toxicol Appl Pharmacol* 2004; 199:142-50.

[213] Dolinoy DC. Epigenetic gene regulation: early environmental exposures. *Pharmacogenomics* 2007; 8:5-10.

[214] Avissar-Whiting M, Veiga KR, Uhl KM, *et al.* Bisphenol A exposure leads to specific microRNA alterations in placental cells. *Reprod Toxicol*; 29:401-6.

[215] vom Saal FS, Akingbemi BT, Belcher SM, *et al.* Chapel Hill bisphenol A expert panel consensus statement: integration of mechanisms, effects in animals and potential to impact human health at current levels of exposure. *Reprod Toxicol* 2007; 24:131-8.

Chapter 2

EFFECTS OF ESTROGEN USE, FOLLICLE-STIMULATING HORMONE AND LUTEINIZING HORMONE ON COGNITIVE TESTS DEMANDING ATTENTION IN POSTMENOPAUSAL WOMEN

Silvia Solís-Ortiz, Elva Pérez-Luque,*
and Ma. Teresa Sepúlveda-Angulo
Departamento de Ciencias Médicas, División de Ciencias de la Salud,
Campus León, Universidad de Guanajuato, Guanajuato, México

INTRODUCTION

Behavioral studies that have evaluated the effects of menopause on some aspects of cognition suggest that certain impairments in cognitive performance are symptomatic of menopause. Cognitive deficits such as poor memory, inability to concentrate, deficits in abstract reasoning, attention and set-shifting flexibility, visuospatial ability, episodic memory and verbal fluency have been reported in middle-aged postmenopausal women [1-3, 4]. Interestingly, differences have not been found in attention, verbal fluency or memory when

* Corresponding author, Silvia Solís-Ortiz, Departamento de Ciencias Médicas, División de Ciencias de la Salud, Campus León, Universidad de Guanajuato, 20 de enero 929, León, Guanajuato, 37320, México. Email: silviasolis17@prodigy.net.mx

comparing cognitive function in late versus early postmenopausal stages [5]. Cognitive decline associated with postmenopause may be due to several factors including hormonal changes [6, 7], normal aging processes [8, 9], age-related changes in dopaminergic neurotransmission [10] and interindividual variations in brain function and cognitive abilities associated with genetic factors [11-13].

Because estrogens have been found to be associated with the maintenance and protection of brain structures in animal models, it is biologically plausible that maintaining high levels of estrogens in postmenopausal women by medication could be protective against cognitive decline. Estrogen replacement therapy (ERT) might be beneficial for the improvement of mood and cognition in menopausal women [14-17]. Estrogen is a multipurpose messenger that can interact with neurotransmitter systems at critical brain nuclei and facilitate neuronal function by affecting gene expression and transmitter-gated ion channels [18]. Estrogen actions on cognition have found support in data that indicate the existence of estrogen receptors in nonreproductive brain structures. The nature of these receptors and the possible mechanisms of action on cognition have been described in many studies [19-21]. Estrogens exert some of their effects through genomic and non-genomic mechanisms [22]. The genomic effects involve the steroid interaction with intracellular receptors and imply the activation of transcription factors [23-25]. The non-genomic process of estrogens is mediated through a subpopulation of the classical estrogen receptors (ERs), estrogen receptors α (ERα) and estrogen receptors β (ERβ), which are located at the plasma membrane and via second messengers with an effect on neuronal excitability [24, 26]. Estrogen receptors are found in the hippocampus, cerebral cortex and amygdala [27-29], which are areas of the brain involved in memory processes, mood and emotion. Moreover, estrogens rapidly increase the number of dendritic spines and synapses in CA1 of the rat hippocampus, which is critical for memory [30, 31], enhancing long-term potentiation in CA1 [32], the production of new cells in the dentate gyrus [33], cholinergic function [34], spatial learning [35] and a number of neurotrophic and neuroprotective effects [36-38].

The results of observational studies that have attempted to link hormone levels and cognitive function in postmenopausal women, however, have been inconclusive. Some studies have reported harmful associations, others have found a protective role, and still others have failed to identify a link between serum estrogen levels and cognitive ability [39, 17]. Some of the inconsistency in the human literature may be explained by methodological differences between studies, such as the characteristics of the population enrolled, the dose or the drug and their routes of administration and methodological issues. However, these differences have failed to convincingly explain discrepancies between studies in this area [40]. Despite the inconsistencies, the diminished postmenopausal production of endogenous estrogen may have a slight negative influence on cognitive abilities and on hormonal replacement therapy as protective.

Changes in scores on neuropsychological tests have been used to assess the possible influence of hormonal replacement therapy during postmen-pause. Because performance on any neuropsychological test requires attention, which is the key to successful information processing, it is necessary to understand attentional performance under the influence of hormone therapy. Attention refers to a process of cognitive control that selects information from a wide range of possible input stimuli and performs an enormous range of possible actions [41]. Most experimental work conducted on the neurobiology of attention is based on the theory of the filter, which states that the central nervous system continuously receives a great amount of stimulation; due to its limited capacity to process all of this information, the system must filter it through a mechanism that allows it to select only those stimuli relevant to perform a task [41]. Attention components include initiation or focusing, sustained attention or vigilance, inhibiting responses to irrelevant stimuli or selective attention, shifting attention [42-44], attentional capacity and response selection over time [45]. At the same time, components of attention are impacted by the overall arousal state of the individual [45].

During the performance of a task that requires a sustained state of alertness, PET scan have shown increased activity in the right frontal and right parietal lobes, whereas the anterior cingulated is quiet, playing a role in target detection. These areas have been proposed as part of a network responsible for maintaining the alert state [46, 47]. In particular, the frontal region has been proposed to be sensitive to the effects of female sex hormones [48, 49].

Attention tests are easily performed by individuals with an intact ability to focus attention, although age [50] and hormonal status may affect this process in women [51-54]. Most studies have compared test scores to evaluate neuropsychological function and its possible relation to estrogen replacement therapy in postmenopausal women. In some cases, this method has provided relevant information but in other cases the findings reported are discrepant. Specific neuropsychological tests that measure sustained attention and the capacity/encoding of attention in an effort to evaluate the effects of the use of estrogens in postmenopausal women have not been sufficiently conclusive. The aim of the current study was to examine the effects of estrogen replacement therapy on processes of attention in healthy postmenopausal women. We hypothesized that measures of sustained attention, attention span and word span would differ depending on estrogen use and that these measures would be correlated with serum hormonal levels.

METHOD

To test this hypothesis we analyzed 50 women who responded to recruitment advertisements. Of the 50 respondents, 30 healthy postmenopausal women volunteers between 48 and 65 years old with an intact uterus were selected based on hormonal state: 15 were users of estrogen replacement therapy for at least 6 months, and 15 were non-users. Female estrogen users took Premarin (0.625 mg), the most widely prescribed conjugated equine estrogen for postmenopausal use, over periods of 6 months to 5 years.

This sample size was calculated to yield an expected power of 0.86 to detect a 10% difference on a cognitive performance task with a two-sided significance level of $\alpha = 0.05$. All of the women were given a medical history interview to assess their health status. To participate in the study, women must have been amenorrheic for at least 12 months and have no history of cardiovascular, metabolic, endocrinological or malignant diseases. None of the participants took any type of medication except estrogens at the time of the study. Incipient dementia was ruled out with the Mini-Mental State Examination (MMSE) [55]. The scores of this test range from 0 to 30, and subjects with dementia generally score below 24. In the present study groups, the MMSE scores ranged from 27 to 30. Participants were tested in a single session by one trained female researcher (between 0900 h and 1100 h). Participants were instructed to abstain from caffeine, alcohol and smoking and to sleep for 8 h on the day prior to testing. This study was approved by the Ethics Committee of the Department of Medical Sciences of the University of Guanajuato for Research on Human Subjects and is in accordance with the Declaration of Helsinki. All subjects provided written informed consent prior to participating in the study.

We used three standard neuropsychological tests to evaluate attention performance, the Continuous Performance Test (sustained attention), the Digit Span Test (attention span), and Sentence Repetition Test (word span). Each test was administered one time during one session, distributed at random. The neuropsychological tests are described below according to the abilities they represent.

Sustained Attention

We used a computerized version of the Continuous Performance Test (CPT) to examine the ability to sustain attention [56]. Performance of the CPT activates the right frontal and parietal lobes [46, 47]. This test has been shown to be sensitive to hormonal changes during menopause [54], and performance is favored by progesterone [53]. This sustained attention test requires the maintenance of a constant level of alertness during the execution of a monotonous task for the detection of a target that is distributed randomly within a sequence of distracters. The sustained attention test consists of 150 alphabet letters displayed continuously in a random sequence, one at a time, for 50 ms on a video screen. The inter-trial interval ranged randomly from 5 to 7 s. The subjects were instructed to perform the test at two different levels of difficulty. In the first level, the letter "S" pattern was selected as the target stimulus, and the subject was asked to press the "enter" button on the keyboard as soon as possible each time the target stimulus was perceived. In the second level, this instruction was maintained, and the subject was asked to press the "enter" button only when the target stimulus was preceded by a specified item, the letter "A", increasing the level of demand for focusing attention. Reaction time, omissions, errors and correct responses were computed.

Attention Span

We used a computerized version of the Digit Span Test [57] to examine attentional capacity. The stimuli used were sequences of numbers presented one by one in the center of a computer screen. The stimuli were presented every 500 ms with a post-interval of 700 ms. The test included two sections. The first section included 7 levels with two sequences of numbers each. At the end of each sequence, the subject was asked to reproduce the sequence in exactly the same order as it was given (forward) by pressing the numeric buttons of the keyboard. Upon completion, the subject pressed the return key. The second section also included 7 levels with two sequences of numbers each. At the end of each sequence, the subject was asked to reproduce the sequence in the reverse order as shown (backward) by pressing the numeric buttons of the keyboard. Upon completion, the subject pressed the return key. The number of sequences replicated forward and backward was computed.

Word Repetition Span

We used a version of the Sentence Repetition Test [58] to examine the attention span for verbal material. The test consisted of reading aloud 64 sentences and reproducing the last word of each sentence in the same order in which they were read. The degree of span was increased after a sequence of 10 sentences. The number of words correctly reproduced was analyzed.

We collected a 10 ml blood sample from participants to measure hormonal levels and to confirm the hormonal status of participants. ELISA was used to determine the 17β-estradiol and progesterone levels. Commercially available radioimmunoassay kits were used to determine luteinizing hormone (LH) and follicle stimulating hormone (FSH) levels.

We performed statistical analyses with STATISTICA for Windows 8 (StatSoft, Inc). Before statistical procedures were applied, the data were tested for a normal distribution using Levene's test. Student's t-test was used to compare the scores of each test, the demographic characteristics and the hormonal levels between estrogen users and non-users. Spearman's correlation test was used to correlate hormone levels with test scores between estrogen users and non-users. Significance was defined as alpha levels of $p < 0.05$.

RESULTS

We did not find significant differences among demographic or clinical variables between estrogen users and non-users in age, schooling, menarche, menopausal years, blood pressure, weight, height, body mass, or pregnancies. The characteristics of the subjects are summarized in Table 1. Estrogen users and non-users showed significant differences in hormone levels. Estradiol ($p = 0.0001$) and estrone ($p = 0.002$) were significantly higher among women using estrogen, whereas levels of LH ($p = 0.0003$) and FSH ($p = 0.00006$) were significantly higher among non-users of estrogen (Table 2).

Table 3 shows the results of attentional performance for the two groups, those using estrogen and non-users. The comparison between means did not reveal a significant difference for any variable on the sustained attention test. At the first difficulty level, the number of correct responses ($p = 0.85$), the number of errors ($p = 0.53$), the number of omissions ($p = 0.78$), and the reaction time ($p = 0.75$) were similar among the women using estrogen and non-users. At the second difficulty level, the number of correct responses ($p = 0.41$), the number of errors ($p = 0.71$), the number of omissions ($p = 0.32$), and the reaction time (p = 0.48) were similar among the women using estrogen and non-users. The comparison between means did not reveal a significant difference for the variables of the attention span test. The number of sequences replicated forward was similar among the women using estrogen and non-users (p = 0.21). The number of sequences replicated backward was similar among the women using estrogen and non-users (p = 0.18). The comparison between means did not reveal a significant difference for the word repetition test. The number of replicated words was similar among women using estrogen and non-users (p = 0.70). We show the results of the correlation between hormonal levels and test scores for the two groups, those using estrogen and non-users, in Table 4. The estradiol levels in women using estrogen were positively correlated with the number of sequences replicated backward (r = 0.56, p <0.05) on the Digit Span Test and with the number of correct responses (r = 0.66, p<0.05) and were negatively correlated with the number of omissions (r = -0.69, p<0.05) at the first level of difficulty on the Sustained Attention Test. The LH levels in women who did not use estrogen were negatively correlated with the reaction time (r = -0.60, p<0.05) at the second level of difficulty on the Sustained Attention Test, whereas the FSH levels were positively correlated with the number of errors (r = 0.53, p<0.05) at the second level of difficulty on the Sustained Attention Test.

Table 1. Estrogen users and non-users characteristics

	Estrogen users Mean ± S.D.	Estrogen non-users Mean ± S.D.	t	p
Age (years)	51.4 ± 4.48	53.4 ± 4.76	-1.184	0.24
Education (years)	9.93 ± 2.40	9.00 ± 2.26	1.093	0.28
Menarche (years)	12.0 ± 1.58	12.3 ± 1.54	-0.467	0.64
Menopause (years)	5.26 ± 4.44	6.93 ± 3.53	-1.136	0.26
Partus	3.33 ± 1.98	4.66 ± 3.31	-1.337	0.19

Table 1. (Continued)

Number of sons	2.66 ± 1.83	3.53 ± 2.47	-1.088	0.28
Weight (kg)	66.3 ± 10.3	64.8 ± 3.70	0.541	0.59
Height (m)	1.54 ± 0.04	1.53 ± 0.04	0.453	0.65
Body mass index (kg/m^2)	27.7 ± 3.27	27.0 ± 2.22	0.711	0.48
Systolic T/A (mmHg)	115 ± 9.81	120 ± 6.23	-1.887	0.06
Diastolic T/A (mmHg)	74.7 ± 4.00	77.6 ± 4.57	-1.867	0.07

p values Student´s t-test.

Table 2. Hormonal levels between estrogen users and non-users

	Estrogen users Mean ± S.D.	Estrogen non-users Mean ± S.D.	t	p
Estradiol (pg/mL)	83.9 ± 66.7	6.38 ± 10.1	4.44	0.0001*
Estrone (pg/mL)	54.0 ± 48.3	10.7 ± 11.3	3.37	0.0020*
LH (mUI/mL)	22.8 ± 15.3	43.9 ± 12.6	-4.12	0.0003*
FSH (mUI/mL)	16.3 ± 10.1	34.9 ± 10.8	-4.67	0.0001*

* $p < 0.05$ Student´s t-test.

Table 3. Neuropsychological performance between estrogen users and non-users

	Estrogen users Mean ± S.D.	Estrogen non-users Mean ± S.D.	t	p
Sustained Attention Test				
Reaction time				
Level 1	449.4 ± 42.6	443.5 ± 57.9	0.317	0.75
Level 2	443.9 ± 63.1	429.0 ± 51.3	0.709	0.48

	Estrogen users Mean $\pm$ S.D.	Estrogen non-users Mean $\pm$ S.D.	t	p
Correct responses				
	Estrogen users Mean $\pm$ S.D.	Estrogen non-users Mean $\pm$ S.D.	t	p
Level 1	34.9 $\pm$ 4.15	35.2 $\pm$ 3.82	-0.183	0.85
Level 2	36.8 $\pm$ 3.07	35.5 $\pm$ 4.99	0.836	0.41
Omissions				
Level 1	5.20 $\pm$ 4.11	4.80 $\pm$ 3.84	0.270	0.78
Level 2	3.20 $\pm$ 3.07	4.73 $\pm$ 3.89	-1.000	0.32
Errors				
Level 1	0.93 $\pm$ 0.88	1.26 $\pm$ 1.83	-0.635	0.53
Level 2	2.33 $\pm$ 3.01	2.80 $\pm$ 3.89	-0.367	0.71
Word Retention Span	26.0 $\pm$ 6.18	25.0 $\pm$ 7.27	0.388	0.70
Attention Span				
Forward	2.80 $\pm$ 1.89	3.53 $\pm$ 1.18	-1.269	0.21
Backforward	2.20 $\pm$ 1.61	2.86 $\pm$ 0.99	-1.360	0.18

p values Student´s t-test.

Table 4. Correlation between hormonal levels and test scores

		Estro.	users			Estro.	Non-users	
Test/ Hormone	Estro.	LH	Estrad.	FSH	Estro.	LH	Estrad.	FSH
Sustained Attention Test								
Reaction time								
Level 1	-0.04	0.13	-0.40	0.25	-0.05	-0.36	-0.37	-0.20
Level 2	-0.30	-0.05	-0.36	-0.07	-0.05	**-0.60***	-0.39	-0.39
Correct responses								
Level 1	0.26	-0.26	**0.66***	-0.41	0.08	0.31	0.25	0.26

Table 4. (Continued)

		Estro. users				Estro. Non-users		
Test/ Hormone	Estro.	LH	Estrad.	FSH	Estro.	LH	Estrad.	FSH
Level 2	-0.03	-0.02	-0.02	0.75	0.18	0.21	0.07	0.26
Omissions								
Level 1	-0.26	0.30	**-0.69***	0.46	-0.12	-0.28	-0.22	-0.25
Level 2	0.03	0.02	0.02	-0.07	-0.39	0.35	-0.40	-0.25
Errors								
Level 1	0.25	-0.03	0.10	-0.21	-0.19	0.02	-0.33	0.19
Level 2	-0.07	0.16	-0.12	0.12	-0.39	0.35	-0.40	**0.53***
Word Retention Span	0.18	0.10	0.21	0.14	0.40	-0.19	0.44	-0.25
Attention Span Forward	0.28	0.14	0.41	-0.10	0.12	0.21	0.30	0.15
Back-forward	0.48	-0.08	**0.56***	-0.38	0.05	0.18	0.20	0.09

* $p < 0.05$ Spearman's Correlation Test.

CONCLUSION

We did not find sufficiently evidence to support the hypothesis that estrogen replacement therapy influences performance on neuropsychological tests that require attentional processes to perform complex cognitive tasks, despite high levels of serum estrogen among estrogen users. Although we did not find quantitative differences in test scores between estrogen users and non-users, some significant correlations identified between hormonal levels and attention tests might be relevant. The women who used estrogens showed high serum estrona and estradiol levels. The maintenance of alertness and sustained attention is crucial to successful information processing. Although many measures can be used to assess sustained attention, the Continuous Performance Test (CPT) is the most frequently used measure for this assessment [59, 60]. In addition to assessing sustained attention, most CPTs assess selective attention and response inhibition for an infrequently occurring target or relevant stimulus [61]. We found that the estrogen levels of women who used estrogen were positively correlated with the number of correct responses and were negatively correlated with the number of omissions indicating that these individuals maintained a sustained state of alertness to execute the test successfully. This result may suggest an influence of estrogen on the brain regions that modulate sustained attention. Sustained attention tests require target detection, orientation, recognition of object identity, working memory and the maintenance of vigilance and selective responses over time. All of these executive functions of attention are attributed to the frontal and parietal lobes [46, 47, 59, 62]. The activating role of estrogen, particularly in the prefrontal cortex where estrogen receptors are located [20], may favor a task in which working memory and concentration are necessary to perceive a relevant external stimulus. The effects of estrogen on the central nervous system and cognition have been reviewed in several studies [15, 19, 20, 21, 49] that have suggested that estrogens play a role in cognition. Estrogen receptors have been identified in the hippocampus, cerebral cortex and amygdala [27, 29], areas involved in cognition and emotion. Our findings are consistent with several studies that show differential effects on attention tests. Postmenopausal women treated with estrogen showed better performance on tests of functions involving the frontal lobe [48, 63] and attention tests [64], and women with low estrogen levels made more errors on a sustained attention test [65]. Animal models have shown that 17-β estradiol administration attenuates deficits in sustained and divided attention in young ovariectomized rats and aged acyclic female rats [66]. However, other studies have not found an association between estrogen use and sustained attention tests in postmenpausal women [67].

We also found that estradiol was associated with better attention span, as indicated by the positive correlation with the number of digits replicated backward. The dissociation between processing speed measured by speed-dependent and short-term capacity reflects the basic dimensions of attention, how fast the attentional system operates, and how much it can process at once. Of course speed and quantity are related; the faster a system can process information, the more information will be processed within a given time [68]. Attentional capacity is measured by span tests that expose the subject to increasingly larger (or smaller, in some formats) amounts of information with instructions to indicate how much of the stimulus is immediately taken in by repeating what was seen or heard or indicating what was grasped in some other type of immediate response [69].

It has been suggested that with advancing age, forward span tends to be stable whereas reversed span shrinks [70]. This would explain our findings. The attentional capacity shown by the women in the present study is correlated with the use of estrogen, suggesting that the brain region that modulates attention may be sensitive to the effects of estrogen. However, others studies have not found an association between the Backward Digits Span test and estradiol or FSH [65, 71]. In contrast, we found that FSH levels were positively correlated with the number of errors on the sustained attention test in female non-users estrogen. Errors were associated with inattention and with decreased vigilance [59]. It has been established that the hormone FSH increases around ovulation [72] and with age [73] and it has been used as a marker of the onset of menopause [74, 75]. Elevated levels of FSH may provide indirect evidence of ovarian failure [76] and are probably related to cognition. A study found that well-preserved cognitive functioning in older women was associated with high endogenous levels of follicle stimulating hormone. These findings indicated that gonadotropins can affect cognitive functioning in older postmenopausal women and that luteinizing hormone and follicle stimulating hormone may exert contrasting effects [77]. We also found that serum LH levels, which become elevated after menopause, were negatively correlated with reaction time on the sustained attention test in female non-users of estrogen. Reaction time is an indicator of arousal state that reflects the vigilance of the individual. Our results partially support a study that found a negative correlation between LH and the number of correct responses on a sustained attention test in a group of postmenopausal women without hormone treatment [54]. Specific receptors for LH have been identified in the cortex, hippocampus, dentate gyrus, hypothalamus, area postrema, cerebellum, glial cells, pituitary gland and in neurons of the spinal cord [78-81]. Some of these areas are involved in cognitive processes. In humans, high levels of LH have been associated with poor memory function and an increased incidence of Alzheimer's [77], and levels of LH have been positively correlated with serum beta amyloidal in older men [82]. Rodent studies have shown that LH is capable of modulating cognitive behavior [83] and in the presence of estradiol is detrimental to cognition [84]. Transgenic mice that over-express LH have shown decreased performance on a hippocampal-associated task compared to aged-matched wild-type animals, indicating that increased LH levels in the presence of functional receptors may be at least partially responsible for cognitive decline after menopause [85]. In summary, our findings suggest that the use of estrogens in healthy postmenpausal women does not seem to substantially influence the prolonged maintenance or the capacity for encoding of attention. These processes are necessary to perform complex tasks that involve memory, language and abstraction. The correlations found between estradiol, FSH and LH levels and attention scores among female estrogens users and non-users indicate a weak relationship that may be relevant to cognition. Future research should focus on the hormones FSH and LH and their impact on human cognition, particularly in middle- aged women.

AUTHOR CONTRIBUTIONS

SSO conceived, designed and performed the study and data analysis and drafted the manuscript. EPL conducted the hormonal analyses. MTSA contributed to data analysis. All authors have read and approved the final manuscript.

ACKNOWLEDGMENTS

This work was supported by following grants: CONACYT Grant 135681-M and a grant from the University of Guanajuato. The authors wish to acknowledge the participation of Rafael Marquez-Rangel in the evaluation of some participants.

REFERENCES

[1] Sullivan, M. E. and Fugate, W. N. (2001). Midlife women's attributions about perceived memory changes: observations from the Seattle Midlife Women's Health Study. *Journal Women's Health Gender Based Medical, 10,* 351–362.

[2] Tivis, L. (1999). Alterations in cognitive function in menopause. In D. B. Seifer, and E. A. Kennard (Eds.), *Menopause: Endocrinology and Management* (pp. 97–110). Totowa NJ: Human Press.

[3] Halbreich, U., Lumley, L. A., Palter, S., Manning, C., Gengo, F. and Joe, S. H. (1995). Possible acceleration of age effects on cognition following menopause. *Journal Psychiatry Research, 29,* 153–163.

[4] Thilers, P. P., Macdonald, S.W., Nilsson, L. G. and Herlitz, A. (2010). Accelerated postmenopausal cognitive decline is restricted to women with normal BMI: longitudinal evidence from the Betula project. *Psychoneuroendocrinology, 35,* 516-524.

[5]   Elsabagh, S., Hartley, D. E. and File, S. E. (2007). Cognitive function in late versus early postmenopausal stage. *Maturitas, 56,* 84-93.

[6]   Sherwin, B. B. (2003). Estrogen and cognitive functioning in women. *Endocrine Reviewer, 24,* 133–151.

[7]   Barrett-Connor, E. and Laughlin, G. A. (2009). Endogenous and exogenous estrogen, cognitive function, and dementia in post-menopausal women: evidence from epidemiologic studies and clinical trials. *Seminars in Reproductive Medicine, 27,* 275–282.

[8]   Bäckman, L., Small, B. J., Wahlin, A. and Larsson, M. (1999). Cognitive functioning in very old age. In F. I. M. Craik, and T. A. Salthouse (Eds.), Handbook of Aging and Cognition: Cognitive functioning in very old age (pp. 499–558). Mahwah, NJ: Erlbaum.

[9]   West, R. L. (1996). An application of prefrontal cortex function theory to cognitive aging. *Psychology Bulletin, 120,* 272–292.

[10]   Bäckman, L., Nyberg, L., Lindenberger, U., Li, S. C. and Farde, L. (2006). The correlative triad among aging, dopamine, and cognition: current status and future prospects. *Neuroscience Biobehavioral Reviewer, 30,* 791–807.

[11]   Krugel, L. K., Biele, G., Mohr, P. N., Li, S. C. and Heekeren, H. R. (2009). Genetic variation in dopaminergic neuromodulation influences the ability to rapidly and flexibly adapt decisions. *Proceedings of National Academy of Sciences of the United States of America, 106,* 17951–17956.

[12]   Erickson, K. I., Kim, J. S., Suever, B. L., Voss, M. W., Francis, B. M. and Kramer A. F. (2008). Genetic contributions to age-related decline in executive function: a 10-year longitudinal study of COMT and BDNF polymorphisms. *Frontiers in Human Neuroscience, 2,* 11.

[13]   Solís-Ortiz, S., Pérez-Luque, E., Morado-Crespo, L. and Gutiérrez-Muñoz, M. (2010). Executive functions and selective attention are favored in middle-aged healthy women carriers of the Val/Val genotype of the catechol-o-methyltransferase gene: a behavioral genetic study. Behavioral and Brain Functions, 6, 67.

[14]   Yaffe, K., Grady, D., Pressman, A. and Cummings, S. (1998). Serum estrogen levels, cognitive performance, and risk of cognitive decline in older community women. *Journal American Geriatric Society, 46,* 816-821.

[15]   Sherwin, B. B. (2003). Estrogen and cognitive functioning in women. *Endocrine Reviewer, 24,* 133–151.

[16] Hogervorst, E., Yaffe, K., Richards, M. and Huppert, F. (2002). Hormone replacement therapy for cognitive function in postmenopausal women. *Cochrane Database Systematic Reviews, 3,* CD003122.

[17] Lethaby, A., Hogervorst, E., Richards, M., Yesufu, A. and Yaffe, K. (2008). Hormone replacement therapy for cognitive function in postmenopausal women. *Cochrane Database of Systematic Reviews, 23,* CD003122.

[18] Fink, G., Sumner, B. E., Rosie, R., Grace, O. and Quinn, J. P. (1996). Estrogen control of central neurotransmission: effect on mood, mental state, and memory. *Cell Molecular Neurobiology, 16,* 325-44

[19] McEwen, B. S., Alves, S. E., Bulloch, K. and Weiland, N. G. (1997). Ovarian steroids and the brain implications for cognition and aging. *Neurology, 48,* S8-S15.

[20] McEwen, B. S. (2001). Estrogens effects on the brain: multiple sites and molecular mechanisms. *Journal of Applied Physiology, 91,* 2765-2801.

[21] Björnström, L. and Sjöberg, M. (2005). Mechanisms of estrogen receptor signaling: convergence of genomic and nongenomic actions on target genes. *Journal of Molecular Endocrinology, 19,* 833-842.

[22] McEwen, B. S. and Alves, S.E. (1999). Estrogen actions in the central nervous system. *Endocrine Reviews, 20,* 279-307.

[23] Lee, S. and McEwen, B. (2001). Neurotrophic and neuroprotective actions of estrogens and their therapeutic implications. *Annual Review of Pharmacology and Toxicology, 41,* 569-591.

[24] McEwen, B. S. (2001). Estrogens effects on the brain: multiple sites and molecular mechanisms. *Journal of Applied Physiology, 91,* 2765-2801.

[25] McEwen, B. S., Akama, K. T., Spencer-Segal, J. L., Milner, T. A. and Waters, E. M. (2012). Estrogen effects on the brain: Actions beyond the hypothalamus via novel mechanisms. *Behavioral Neuroscience, 126,* 4-16

[26] Razandi, M., Pedram, A., Greene, G. L. and Levin, E. R. (1999). Cell membrane and nuclear estrogen receptor (Ers) originate from a single transcript: studies of ERα and ERβ expressed in Chinese hamster ovary cells. *Journal of Molecular Endocrinology, 13,* 307-319.

[27] Register, T. C., Shively, C. A. and Lewis, C. E. (1998). Expression of estrogen receptor alpha and beta transcripts in female monkey hippocampus and hypothalamus. *Brain Research Journal, 788,* 320-322.

[28] Blurton-Jones, M. M., Roberts, J. A. and Tuszynski, M. H. (1999). Estrogen receptor inmunoreactivity in the adult primate brain: neuronal distribution and association with p75, trkA, and choline acetyltransferase. *The Journal of Comparative Neurology*, 405, 529-542.

[29] Gundlah, C., Kohama, S. G., Mirkes, S. J., Garyfallou, V. T., Urbanski, H. F. and Bethea, C. L. (2000). Distribution of estrogen receptor beta (ERbeta) mRNA in hypothalamus, midbrain and temporal lobe of spayed macaque: continued expression with hormone replacement. *Brain Research Molecular Brain Research, 76*, 191-204.

[30] Woolley, C. S. (1998). Estrogen-mediated structural and functional synaptic plasticity in the female rat hippocampus. *Hormones and Behavior, 3,* 140-148.

[31] Woolley, C. S. (1999). Electrophysiological and cellular effects of estrogen on neuronal function. *Critical Reviews in Clinical Neurobiology*, 13, 1-20.

[32] Cordoba Montoya, D. M. and Carrer, H. F. (1997). Estrogen facilitates induction of long term potentiation in the hippocampus of awake rats. *Brain Research Journal, 778,* 430-438.

[33] Tenapat, P., Hastings, N. B., Reeves, A. J. and Gould, E. (1999). Estrogen stimulates a transient increase in the number of the new neurons in the dentate gyrus of the adult female rat. *Journal of Neuroscience, 19,* 5792-5801.

[34] Gibbs, R. B. (1998). Impairment of basal forebrain cholinergic neurons associated with aging and long-term loss of ovarian function. *Experimental Neurology, 151,* 289-302.

[35] Frye, C. A., Duffy, C. K. and Walf, A. A. (2007). Estrogens and progestins enhance spatial learning of intact and ovariectomized rats in the objects placement task. *Neurobiology of Learning and Memory, 88,* 208-216.

[36] Wise, P. M., Smith, M. J., Dubal, D. B., Wilson, M. E., Krajnak, K. M. and Rosewell, K. L. (1999). Neuroendocrine influences and repercussions of the menopause. *Endocrine Reviews, 20,* 243-248.

[37] Brinton, R. D., Chen, S., Montoya, M., Hsieh, D., Minaya, J., Kim, J. and Chu, H. P. (2000). The women´s health initiative estrogen replacement therapy is neurotrophic and neuroprotective. *Neurobiology of Aging, 21,* 475-496.

[38] Green, P. S. and Simpkins, J. W. (2000). Neuroprotective effects of estrogen: potential mechanisms of action. *International Journal of Developmental Neuroscience: The Official Journal of the International Society for Developmental Neuroscience, 18,* 347-358.

[39] Craig, M. C., Maki, P. M. and Murphy, D. G. (2005). The Women's Health Initiative Memory Study: findings and implications for treatment. *Lancet Neurology, 4,* 190-194.

[40] Sherwin, B.B. (2012). Estrogen and cognitive functioning in women: Lessons we have learned. *Behavioral Neuroscience, 126,* 123-127.

[41] Broadbent, D. B. (1971). Decision and Stress. London: Academic Press.

[42] Denckla, M. B. (1996). Biological correlates of learning and attention: what is relevant to learning disabilities and attention deficit hyperactivity disorder? *Journal of Developmental and Behavioral Pediatrics, 17,* 114-119.

[43] Mirsky, A. F. (1987). Behavioral and psychophysiological markers of disordered attention. *Environmental Health Perspectives, 74,* 191-199.

[44] Mirsky, A. F., Anthony, B. J., Duncan, C. C., Ahearn, M. B. and Kellam, S. G. (1991). Analysis of the elements of attention: a neuropsychological approach. *Neuropsychology Review, 12,* 109-145.

[45] Cohen, R. A. and O´Donnell, B. F. (1993). Models and mechanisms of attention: A summary. In R.A. Cohen (Ed.). *The Neuropsychology of Attention* (pp. 177-188). New York: Plenum.

[46] Posner, M. I. and Raichle, M. E. (1994). Networks of Attention. In M. I. Posner, and M. E. Raichle, (Eds.), *Images of Mind.* (pp. 153-179). New York: A Scientific American Library.

[47] Fan, J. and Posner, M. (2004). Human attentional networks. *Psychiatrische Praxis, 31(S2),* 10-4.

[48] Keenan, P. A., Ezzat, W. H., Ginsburg, K. and Moore, G. J. (2001). Prefrontal cortex as the site of estrogen´s effect on cognition. *Psychoneuroendocrinology, 26,* 577-590.

[49] Maki, P. M. (2005). Estrogen effects on the hippocampus and frontal lobes. *International Journal Fertility Women's Medicine, 50,* 67-71.

[50] Sieroff, E. and Piquard, A. (2004). Attention and aging. *Psychologie and Neuropsychiatrie du Vieillissement, 2,* 257-69.

[51] Sommer, B. (1992). Cognitive performance and the menstrual cycle. In J.T.E. Richardson (Ed.), *Cognition and the Menstrual Cycle.* (pp. 39-56). New York: Springer-Verlag.

[52] Smith, Y. R., Giordani, B. G., Lajiness-O´Neill, R. and Zubieta, J. K. (2001). Long-term estrogen replacement is associated with improved nonverbal memory and attentional measures in postmenopausal women. *Fertility and Sterility, 76,* 1101-1107.

[53] Solis-Ortiz, S. and Corsi-Cabrera, M. (2008). Sustained attention is favored by progesterone during early luteal phase and visuo-spatial memory by estrogens during ovulatory phase in young women. *Psychoneuroendocrinology, 33,* 989-998.

[54] Sepúlveda-Angulo, M. T., Pérez-Luque, E. and Solís-Ortiz, S. (2009). Atención sostenida asociada con hormonas ováricas en mujeres en la premenopausia y posmenopausia. *Revista Chilena de Neuropsicología, 4,* 149-159.

[55] Folstein, M. F., Folstein, S. F. and McHugh, P. R. (1975). Mini-mental state: A practical method for grading the cognitive state of patients for the clinician. *Journal Psychiatry Research, 12,* 189–198.

[56] Rosvold, H., Mirsky, A., Sarason, I., Bransome, E. D. and Beck, L. H. (1956). A continuous performance test of brain damage. *Journal of Consulting Psychology, 20,* 343-350.

[57] Weschler, D. (1981). Weschler Adult Intelligence Scale-Revised. New York: Psychological Corporation.

[58] Yáñez, G., Bernal, J., Harmony, T., Marosi, E. and Rodríguez, M. (2002). Batería Neuropsicológica para Niños con Trastornos del Aprendizaje de la Lectura (BNTAL): Obtención de Normas. Revista Latina de Pensamiento y Lenguaje y Neuropsicología Latina, *10,* 2.

[59] Bearden, T. S., Cassisi, J. E. and White, J. N. (2004). Electrophysiological correlates of vigilance during a continous performance test in healthy adults. *Applied Neurophysiology Biofeedback, 29,*75-88.

[60] DuPaul, G. L., Anasropoulos, A. D., Shelton, T. L., Guevremont, D. C. and Metevia, L. (1992). Multimethod assesment of attention deficit hyperactivity disorder: The diagnostic utility of clinic-based tests. *Journal of Clinical Child Psychology, 21,* 394- 402.

[61] Riccio, C. A., Reynolds, C. R. and Lowe, P. A. (2001). Clinical Applications of Continuous Performance Tests. New York: Wiley.

[62] Riccio, C. A., Reynolds, C. R., Lowe, P, and Moore, J. J. (2002). The Continuous Performance Test: a window on the neural substrates for attention? *Archives of Clinical Neuropsychology, 17,* 235-272.

[63] Joffe, H., Hall, J. E., Gruber, S., Sarmiento, I. A., Lee, B. A., Cohen, S., Yurgehun-Todd, D. and Nartin, K. A. (2006). Estrogen therapy selectively enhances prefrontal cognitive processes: a randomized, double-blind, placebo-controlled study with functional magnetic resonance imaging in perimenopausal and recently posmenopausal women. *Menopause, 13,* 411-422.

[64] Wroolie, T. E., Kenna, H. A., Williams, K. E., Powers, B. N., Holcomb, M., Khaylis, A. and Rasgon, N. L. (2011). Differences in verbal memory performance in postmenopausal women receiving hormone therapy: 17β-estradiol versus conjugated equine estrogens. *American Journal Geriatric Psychiatry, 19,* 792-802.

[65] Portin, R., Polo-Kantola, P., Polo, O., Koskinen, T., Revonsuo, A., Irjala, K. and Erkkola, R. (1999). Serum estrogen level, attention, memory and other cognitive functions in middle-aged women. *Climateric, 2,*115-123.

[66] Barnes, P., Staal, V., Muir, J. and Good, M. A. (2006). 17-Beta estradiol administration attenuates deficits in sustained and divided attention in young ovariectomized rats and aged acyclic female rats. *Behavioral Neuroscience, 120,* 1225-1234.

[67] Krug, R., Mölle, M., Dodt, C., Fehm, H. L. and Born, J. (2006). Acute influences of estrogen and testosterone on divergent and convergent thinking in postmenopausal women. *Neuropsychopharmacology, 28,* 1538-1545.

[68] Shum, D. H. K., McFarland, K. A., and Bain, J. D. (1990). Construct validity of eight tests of attention: Comparison of normal and closed heard injured samples. *The Clinical Neuropsychologist, 4,* 151-162.

[69] Lesak, M. D. (1995). Neuropsychological Assessment. (Third Edition, pp. 335-384). New York: Oxford University Press.

[70] Hayslip, B., and Sterns, H. L. (1979). Age differences in relationships between crystallized and fluid intelligence and problem solving. *Journal of Gerontology, 34,* 404-414.

[71] Luetters, C., Huang, M. H., Seeman, T., Buckwalter, G., Meyer, P. M, Avis, N. E., Sternfeld, B., Johnston, J. M. and Greendale, G. A. (2007). Menopause transition stage and endogenous estradiol and follicle-stimulating hormone levels are not related to cognitive performance: cross-sectional results from the study of women's health across the nation (SWAN). *Journal Womens Health, 16,* 331-344.

[72] Marshall, J. C. (2001). Hormonal regulation of menstrual cycle and mechanisms of ovulation. In J, Leslie, L. J., De Groot, and L. J. Jamerson (Eds.), *Endocrinology* (Fourth Edition). Philadelphia: W. B. Saunders Company.

[73] Backer, L. C., Ruvin, C. S., Marcus, M., Kieszak, S. M. and Schober, S. E. (1999). Serum follicle-stimulating hormone and luteinizing hormone levels in women aged 35-60 in the U.S. population: the Third National Health and Nutrition Examination Survey (NHANES III, 1988-1994). *Menopause, 6,* 29-35.

[74] Burger, H. G. (1994). Diagnostic role of follicle-stimulating hormone (FSH) measurements during the menopausal transition--an analysis of FSH, oestradiol and inhibin. *European Journal Endocrinology, 130,* 38-42.

[75] Randolph, J. F. Jr., Crawford, S., Dennerstein, L., Cain, K., Harlow, S. D., Little, R., Mitchell, E. S., Nan, B., Taffe, J. and Yosef, M. (2006). The value of follicle-stimulating hormone concentration and clinical findings as markers of the late menopausal transition. *Journal Clinical Endocrinology Metabolism, 91,* 3034-3040.

[76] Santoro, N. and Tortoriello, D. V. (1999). Endocrinology of the Climateric. In D.B. Seifer, and E.A. Kennard (Eds.), *Menopause: Endocrinology and Management* (pp. 21-34).Totowa, New Jersey: Human Press.

[77] Rodrigues, M. A., Verdile, G., Foster, J. K., Hogervorst, E., Joesbury, K., Dhaliwal, S., Corder, E. H., Laws, S. M., Hone, E., Prince, R., Devine, A., Mehta, P., Beilby, J., Atwood, C. S. and Martins, R. N. (2008). Gonadotropins and cognition in older women. *Journal Aizheimer´s Disease, 13,* 267-274.

[78] Lei, Z. M., Rao, C.V., Kornyei, J. L., Licht, P. and Hiatt, E. S. (1993). Novel expression of human chorionic gonadotropin/luteinizing hormone receptor gene in brain. *Endocrinology, 132,* 2262-2270.

[79] Hamalainen, T., Poutanen, M. and Huhtaniemi, I. (1999). Age- and sex-specific promoter function of a 2-kilobase 5′-flanking sequence of the murine luteinizing hormone receptor gene in transgenic mice. *Endocrinology, 140,* 5322–5329.

[80] Lei, Z. M. (2001). Neural actions of LH and human chorionic. *Seminars in Reproductive Medicine, 19,* 103-109.

[81] Apaja, P. M., Harju, K. T., Aatsinki, J. T., Petaja-Repo, U. E. and Rajaniemi, H. J. (2004). Identification and structural characterization of the neuronal luteinizing hormone receptor associated with sensory systems. *Journal Biological Chemistry, 279,* 1899–1906.

[82] Verdile, G., Yeap, B. B., Clarnette, R. M., Dhaliwal, S., Burkhardt, M. S., Chubb, S. A., De Ruyck, K., Rodrigues, M., Mehta, P. D., Foster, J. K., Bruce, D. G. and Martins, R. N. (2008). Luteinizing hormone levels are positively correlated with plasma amyloid-beta protein levels in elderly men. *Journal Alzheimers Disease, 14,* 201–208.

[83] Lukacs, H., Hiatt, E. S., Lei, Z. M. and Rao, C. V. (1995). Peripheral and intracerebroventricular administration of human chorionic gonadotropin alters several hippocampus-associated behaviors in cycling female rats. *Hormonal Behavior, 29,* 42-58.

[84] Berry, A., Tomidokoro, Y., Ghiso, J. and Thornton, J. (2008). Human chorionic gonadotropin (a luteinizing hormone homologue) decreases spatial memory and increases brain amyloid-beta levels in female rats. *Hormone Behavior, 54,*143–152.

[85] Casadesus, G., Webber, K. M., Atwood, C. S., Pappolla, M. A., Perry, G., Bowen, R. L. and Smith, M. A. (2006). Luteinizing hormone modulates cognition and amyloid deposition in Alzheimer APP transgenic mice. *Biochimica et Biophysica Acta, 176,* 447-452.

In: Estrogens
Editors: V. Thompson and A. Watson

ISBN 978-1-62081-747-6
© 2012 Nova Science Publishers, Inc.

Chapter 3

THE ROLE OF ESTROGENS IN OSTEOARTHRITIS AND INFLAMMATION

Marta Martín Millán[1], and Santos Castañeda[2]*
[1]Department of Internal Medicine, IFIMAV, Hospital Universitario
Marqués de Valdecilla, Santander, Cantabria, Spain
[2]Department of Rheumatology, IIS-Princesa, Hospital Universitario
de La Princesa, Madrid, Spain

ABSTRACT

It has been observed that osteoarthritis is more prevalent once menopause is established, which has suggested the link between estrogens and healthy joints. In addition, deletion of estrogen receptors in female mice results in cartilage damage, osteophytosis and changes in subchondral bone of adult skeleton, suggesting that estrogen, through its receptor, has a protective role on the maintenance of normal joints. Furthermore, it has been postulated that acute loss of estrogens increases the levels of reactive oxygen species and activates nuclear factor-kB and cytokine production, which indicates that estrogens have also anti-inflammatory properties.

Pro-inflammatory cytokine expression has been shown to be attenuated by estrogen replacement. The ability of estrogen to attenuate

---

* Corresponding author: Marta Millán, Department of Internal Medicine, IFIMAV, Hospital Universitario Marqués de Valdecilla, Avenida de Valdecilla s/n, 39008-Santander, Cantabria, Spain. E-mail: martinmma@unican.es. Telephnone: + 34. 942 201990.

the effects of oxidative stress is mediated, in part, by mechanisms that do not require stimulation of the nuclear-initiated actions of sex steroids. In spite of the negative effect of estrogen replacement reported in 2003 by the Women's Health Initiative (WHI) results, several studies published afterwards have explored the potential protective effect of estrogen supplementation in animal models and demonstrated possible reasons why these actions may justify a beneficial role of estrogens in degenerative joint disease.

In this chapter, we will revise the effects of estrogens in healthy and osteoarthritic or inflamed joints, especially in postmenopausal women.

Keywords: Estrogens, osteoarthritis, bone, inflammation

INTRODUCTION

Estrogens regulate many physiological processes, including normal cell growth, development, and tissue-specific gene regulation in the reproductive tract, the brain, the immune system, and the cardiovascular and skeletal systems [1, 2].

The biological actions of estrogens are mediated by binding to one of two specific estrogen receptors (ERs), ERα or ERβ, located mainly in the cytoplasm [1]. For several years, it was thought that there was only one type of receptor, now known as ERα. However, in the 90's several laboratories independently discovered another protein, encoded by a different gene, located in another different chromosome which was called ERβ [3-5]. Both receptors are expressed in a variety of tissues throughout the body, but in different proportions.

ERα is highly expressed in classical estrogen target tissues such as the uterus, placenta, pituitary and cardiovascular system, whereas ERβ is more abundant in the ventral prostate, urogenital tract, ovarian follicles, lung, and immune system.

However, both ERs are co-expressed in the mammary gland, bone, and certain regions of the brain. In joint tissues [6], both ER types are expressed by the chondrocytes [7], subchondral bone cells [8], synoviocytes [9], ligament fibroblasts [10] and myoblasts [11] in humans and other species. Nevertheless, ERα is predominant in cortical bone and ERβ predominates in cartilage, cancellous bone and synovium [9, 12].

ESTROGEN RECEPTORS STRUCTURE AND CHARACTERISTICS

The two receptors have the typical structure of the nuclear receptor family which consists of six regions, designated with letters from A to F. The C domain is a highly conserved region also known as the DNA binding domain (DBD). It recognizes sequences of 13 bp (5'GGTCAnnnTGACC3 '), named as estrogen response element (ERE), and located in the promoter of the target genes [13]. The D domain is a less conserved region, whose flexibility allows the protein to fold up easily. The C-terminal domain includes the ligand binding domain (LBD), which is where the ligand binds to its receptor. This domain also contains a transactivation region, known as AF-2, which is responsible for recruiting co-activators or repressors depending on the ligand bonded [14]. The F domain varies in length, depending on the species, and it is not directly involved in ligand binding or transcriptional activation, but modulates receptor activity [15].

The N-terminal region is the most variable among family members, both in size and amino acid sequences. It contains a transactivation region, called AF-1, which unlike AF-2 it is ligand independent. Both AF-1 and AF-2 regions can activate transcription, independently or synergistically. The N-terminus contains 14 serine residues which can be phosphorylated by a variety of protein kinases [16-18]. It is still unknown the functional importance of post-translational modification of nuclear receptors, but it is thought that phosphorylation of these serine residues might be involved in modulating the activity of AF-1, by means of interaction with co-regulatory elements.

The resulting conformation obtained once ligand has bonded to the ER will determine the type of regulator that will be recruited. Binding of agonists promotes interaction with co-activators, while binding of antagonists induces the interaction with co-repressors.

ERs control gene transcription through at least three well documented mechanisms: direct DNA binding through the EREs, indirect DNA binding through protein-protein interactions with other transcription factors, and through an extranuclear mode by the pool of ER localized at the cellular membrane [19-22]. ERs at the cell membrane can activate kinases mediating phosphorylation of transcription factors, which once they are phosphorylated, can be translocated to the nucleus and induce transcription of their target genes. The three mechanisms exist together in each cell of the organism.

However, there is a balance among them and the prevalence of one upon the other is what determines the final cellular outcome.

Estrogen was originally thought to be exclusively a sexual hormone whose task was the development of the reproductive system. However, during the past 30 years our understanding of its physiological functions has improved. What we know now is that estrogens, through both, direct and indirect mechanisms on different cell types exert a broad spectrum of pleiotropic effects in non-sexual tissues, and that loss of estrogen is involved in many age related conditions. Yet, its precise molecular mechanism remains often not fully understood.

ESTROGEN ON INFLAMMATION

Inflammation is a critical component in several inflammatory and autoimmune diseases such as multiple sclerosis, inflammatory bowel disease, rheumatoid arthritis (RA), systemic lupus erythematosus (SLE), and in a minor degree in osteoarthritis and atherosclerosis, and almost all these disorders mainly affect women. Many players, such as B and T lymphocytes, antigen-presenting cells, monocyte/macrophages, new vessels formation, adhesion molecules, cytokines production and oxygen radicals can contribute to the development of an inflammatory environment. The global effect of estrogens on inflammation will depend on estrogens influence not only on the key players implicated in a particular inflammatory disorder, but also on the cells of the target tissues involved.

ESTROGEN AND AUTOIMMUNE DISEASES: RHEUMATOID ARTHRITIS AND SYSTEMIC LUPUS ERYTHEMATOSUS

Regarding autoimmune diseases, we can distinguish two major stages in the evolution of these diseases: an initiation phase, generally asymptomatic and which starts, depending of the process, until 10 years earlier than the disease outbreak, and a symptomatic phase, which reflects the location of the auto-antigens in a particular tissue. During the first one, T and B lymphocytes and antigen-presenting cells play an important role on auto-reactive T and B cells clonal expansion. Since the influence of estrogens on these players is different from other cell types, estradiol (E_2) have opposite roles depending on the involved cells [23, 24].

Experiments performed *in vitro* and in animal models indicated that estrogens stimulate autoantibody production by B cells, in part, by inhibiting T cells suppression of B cells. In contrast, high levels of E_2 induce a down-regulation of B-lymphocyte lineage in the bone marrow. Therefore, if B cells are the main players in a given autoimmune disease, E_2 would induce the disorder when autoaggressive B-cells are already developed, while chronically elevated E_2 would blunt the initiation of the disease. These data might explain why those B cell-dependent diseases, such as SLE, are developed in women during either their reproductive years or during late-after pregnancy [24].

On the other hand, if tissue-destructive T cells play the most important role, the onset of the disease will be delayed to the late reproductive or postmenopausal period, when E_2 has already declined and T cell autoimmunity is not attenuated any more [24].

Naïve T cells differentiate into either Th1 or Th2, depending on the cytokines secreted by dendritic cells in response to a specific antigenic challenge. Th1 lymphocytes are known as a well established component of the

RA. Th1 secretes interferon gamma (IFNɣ) and lymphotoxin, promoting cell-mediated immunity to intracellular pathogens. By contrast, Th2 lymphocytes tend to secrete interleukins 4 and 5 (IL-4 and IL-5), which function in allergic reactions and humoral immunity to parasites [25]. Those latter lymphocytes are the ones typically involved in SLE disease. High levels of estrogens suppress the Th1-mediated responses and stimulate Th2-mediated immunologic responses. Th2 cells, unlike Th1 cells, produce mostly IL-4, -5, -10 and -13 to promote IgG, IgA, and IgE antibody isotype responses, which is why Th1-mediated diseases, such as RA, tend to improve during pregnancy while Th2-mediated diseases, such as SLE, tend to worsen [26].

ESTROGEN AND OSTEOARTHRITIS

Osteoarthritis (OA) is a disease commonly seen in postmenopausal women. The prevalence of OA is higher among women than men and the prevalence in the woman increases clearly after menopause. In fact, a nationwide population survey showed that radiographic OA is 3 times more common among 45-64 year-old-women compared to their male peers [27, 28].

    Marta Martín Millán and Santos Castañeda

Moreover, OA is also more symptomatic in the woman with the same degree of radiographic damage.

The dramatic rise in OA prevalence among postmenopausal women suggests a link between OA and loss of ovarian function. Different studies have provided compelling information on the relevant effects of estrogen deficiency on joint components in cell culture, animal models or humans. Although much of the attention has focused on the effects of estrogen on articular cartilage, estrogen deficiency also affects other joint tissues during the course of OA, such as the subchondral bone, synovial lining, ligaments and the joint capsule [6]. This association indicates a potential protective role for estrogens against the development of OA. Indeed, recent *in vitro, in vivo,* genetic and clinical studies have shed further light on these issues.

Animal models have shown that ovariectomy (OVX) can induce joint damage, and ERα knockout animals develop higher number and larger osteophytes, as well as thinner lateral subchondral plate [29, 30]. Furthermore, lack of estrogens also increases subchondral bone remodeling, finally inducing osteoarthritis changes. However, results obtained from the models described above can make difficult the interpretation of some data, regarding whether the effect of estrogen deprivation on joints impairment is due to the absence of the hormone itself, or, on the other hand, due to an indirect effect derived from the subchondral bone loss [31].

For this purpose, the rabbit has been proposed as an appropriate model to perform this kind of studies [31]. In this line, Castañeda et al has shown that OVX rabbits did not suffer such a bone mass decline and he has proposed this animal, as a model to study the direct effect of estrogen on cartilage [31, 32]. Interestingly, these authors found mild abnormalities in joint structure, as well as higher Mankin scores, in mature OVX rabbits which did not develop significant changes on subchondral bone mineral density (BMD) with respect to their controls, indicating that estrogens have a protective effect on joint cartilage through both direct and indirect actions [31].

In vitro studies have demonstrated that the direct chondro-protective role of estrogen might be in part by inducing glycosaminoglycan synthesis, which is an important component of connective tissue [33]. E_2 also inhibits cyclo-oxigenase-2 mRNA expression in bovine articular chondrocytes as well as in other tissues, and this fact has been related with protection against reactive oxygen species-induced chondrocyte damage [34, 35].

By contrast, some authors postulate that estrogen could also have a deleterious effect on the chondrocyte metabolism. This statement is based on the data found in young OVX rabbits who received either systemic estrogen replacement or intra-articular estrogen administration. Unexpectedly, those animals exhibited impairment of the joint lesions. At cellular level, it has been shown that high doses of estrogens have an effect on IL1β-stimulated proteoglycan degradation and metalloproteinase production. Therefore, we can conclude that both high and low levels of estrogen can be deleterious for the normal balance of the joints, and the final effect depends on the estradiol concentration at the cartilage microenvironment.

The data available in humans are also contradictory. In this way, polymorphisms in the human ERα gene and radiographic knee OA have been studied in different populations with paradoxical results. Observational studies, however, show the beneficial effect of estrogen replacement in some kind of OA, and that estrogen supplementation decreases the severity of the OA, especially at the hip location. By contrast, a recent study indicates that estrogen induces temporo-mandibular joint inflammation, via NF-kB pathway, in a dose dependent manner [36]. All these observations and data point out that both concentration of estrogen and cartilage location should be taking into account to understand the dual effect of estrogen on chondrocyte homeostasis. Moreover, addition of progestagens to estrogens, in the hormone replacement therapy, could counteract the beneficial effects of estrogens alone on cartilage [37].

CONCLUSION

There are no doubts about the beneficial anti-inflammatory effects of estrogens in many disorders. However, there are several aspects, such as the immune stimuli involved, the target organ or the reproductive status, that should be taken into account when estrogen replacement is administrated. There are still many questions regarding what the optimal concentration which promotes positive effects on joint tissues is, and the appropriate timing of estrogens administration in relation to the course of the disorders that should be addressed in future research.

COMPETING INTERESTS

The authors declare that they have not competing interests in the preparation of this manuscript.

REFERENCES

[1] Pettersson K, Gustafsson JA. Role of estrogen receptor beta in estrogen action. *Annu. Rev. Physiol.* 2001;63:165-92.

[2] Couse JF, Korach KS. Estrogen receptor null mice: what have we learned and where will they lead us? Endocr.Rev. 1999;20(3):358-417.

[3] Kuiper GG, Enmark E, Pelto-Huikko M, Nilsson S, Gustafsson JA. Cloning of a novel receptor expressed in rat prostate and ovary. *Proc. Natl. Acad. Sci. U.S.A* 1996;93(12):5925-30.

[4] Tremblay GB, Tremblay A, Copeland NG, Gilbert DJ, Jenkins NA, Labrie F et al. Cloning, chromosomal localization, and functional analysis of the murine estrogen receptor beta. *Mol. Endocrinol.* 1997; 11(3): 353-65.

[5] Mosselman S, Polman J, Dijkema R. ER beta: identification and characterization of a novel human estrogen receptor. *FEBS Lett.* 1996; 392(1): 49-53.

[6] Roman-Blas JA, Castaneda S, Largo R, Herrero-Beaumont G. Osteoarthritis associated with estrogen deficiency. *Arthritis Res.Ther.* 2009; 11(5):241.

[7] Ushiyama T, Ueyama H, Inoue K, Ohkubo I, Hukuda S. Expression of genes for estrogen receptors alpha and beta in human articular chondrocytes. *Osteoarthritis. Cartilage.* 1999;7(6):560-6.

[8] Braidman IP, Hainey L, Batra G, Selby PL, Saunders PT, Hoyland JA. Localization of estrogen receptor beta protein expression in adult human bone. *J. Bone Miner. Res.* 2001;16(2):214-20.

[9] Dietrich W, Haitel A, Holzer G, Huber JC, Kolbus A, Tschugguel W. Estrogen receptor-beta is the predominant estrogen receptor subtype in normal human synovia. *J. Soc. Gynecol. Investig.* 2006;13(7):512-7.

[10] Sciore P, Frank CB, Hart DA. Identification of sex hormone receptors in human and rabbit ligaments of the knee by reverse transcription-polymerase chain reaction: evidence that receptors are present in tissue from both male and female subjects. *J. Orthop. Res.* 1998;16(5):604-10.

[11] Kahlert S, Grohe C, Karas RH, Lobbert K, Neyses L, Vetter H. Effects of estrogen on skeletal myoblast growth. *Biochem. Biophys. Res. Commun.* 1997;232(2):373-8.

[12]   Bord S, Horner A, Beavan S, Compston J. Estrogen receptors alpha and beta are differentially expressed in developing human bone. *J. Clin. Endocrinol. Metab.* 2001;86(5):2309-14.

[13]   Driscoll MD, Sathya G, Muyan M, Klinge CM, Hilf R, Bambara RA. Sequence requirements for estrogen receptor binding to estrogen response elements. *J. Biol. Chem.* 1998;273(45):29321-30.

[14]   Pike AC. Lessons learnt from structural studies of the oestrogen receptor. *Best. Pract. Res. Clin. Endocrinol. Metab.* 2006;20(1):1-14.

[15]   Koide A, Zhao C, Naganuma M, Abrams J, Deighton-Collins S, Skafar DF et al. Identification of regions within the F domain of the human estrogen receptor alpha that are important for modulating transactivation and protein-protein interactions. *Mol. Endocrinol.* 2007;21(4):829-42.

[16]   Weigel NL, Zhang Y. Ligand-independent activation of steroid hormone receptors. *J. Mol. Med.* 1998;76(7):469-79.

[17]   Britton DJ, Scott GK, Schilling B, Atsriku C, Held JM, Gibson BW et al. A novel serine phosphorylation site detected in the N-terminal domain of estrogen receptor isolated from human breast cancer cells. *J. Am. Soc. Mass Spectrom.* 2008;19(5):729-40.

[18]   Smith CL. Cross-talk between peptide growth factor and estrogen receptor signaling pathways. *Biol. Reprod.* 1998;58(3):627-32.

[19]   Coleman KM, Dutertre M, El Gharbawy A, Rowan BG, Weigel NL, Smith CL. Mechanistic differences in the activation of estrogen receptor-alpha (ER alpha)- and ER beta-dependent gene expression by cAMP signaling pathway(s). *J. Biol. Chem.* 2003;278(15):12834-45.

[20]   Hall JM, Couse JF, Korach KS. The multifaceted mechanisms of estradiol and estrogen receptor signaling. *J. Biol. Chem.* 2001;276(40): 36869-72.

[21]   Pedram A, Razandi M, Levin ER. Nature of functional estrogen receptors at the plasma membrane. *Mol. Endocrinol.* 2006;20(9):1996-2009.

[22]   Razandi M, Oh P, Pedram A, Schnitzer J, Levin ER. ERs associate with and regulate the production of caveolin: implications for signaling and cellular actions. *Mol. Endocrinol.* 2002;16(1):100-15.

[23]   Cutolo M, Capellino S, Straub RH. Oestrogens in rheumatic diseases: friend or foe? *Rheumatology.*(Oxford) 2008;47 Suppl 3:iii2-iii5.

[24]   Straub RH. The complex role of estrogens in inflammation. *Endocr. Rev.* 2007; 28(5):521-74.

[25] Romagnani S. Regulation of the T cell response. *Clin. Exp. Allergy* 2006; 36(11):1357-66.

[26] Munoz-Valle JF, Vazquez-Del Mercado M, Garcia-Iglesias T, Orozco-Barocio G, Bernard-Medina G, Martinez-Bonilla G et al. T(H)1/T(H)2 cytokine profile, metalloprotease-9 activity and hormonal status in pregnant rheumatoid arthritis and systemic lupus erythematosus patients. *Clin. Exp. Immunol.* 2003;131(2):377-84.

[27] Srikanth VK, Fryer JL, Zhai G, Winzenberg TM, Hosmer D, Jones G. A meta-analysis of sex differences prevalence, incidence and severity of osteoarthritis. *Osteoarthritis. Cartilage.* 2005;13(9):769-81.

[28] Lawrence RC, Helmick CG, Arnett FC, Deyo RA, Felson DT, Giannini EH et al. Estimates of the prevalence of arthritis and selected musculoskeletal disorders in the United States. *Arthritis Rheum.* 1998; 41(5):778-99.

[29] Ma HL, Blanchet TJ, Peluso D, Hopkins B, Morris EA, Glasson SS. Osteoarthritis severity is sex dependent in a surgical mouse model. *Osteoarthritis. Cartilage.* 2007;15(6):695-700.

[30] Sniekers YH, van Osch GJ, Ederveen AG, Inzunza J, Gustafsson JA, van Leeuwen JP et al. Development of osteoarthritic features in estrogen receptor knockout mice. *Osteoarthritis. Cartilage.* 2009;17(10):1356-61.

[31] Castaneda S, Largo R, Calvo E, Bellido M, Gomez-Vaquero C, Herrero-Beaumont G. Effects of estrogen deficiency and low bone mineral density on healthy knee cartilage in rabbits. *J. Orthop. Res.* 2010; 28 (6): 812-8.

[32] Castaneda S, Calvo E, Largo R, Gonzalez-Gonzalez R, de la PC, Diaz-Curiel M et al. Characterization of a new experimental model of osteoporosis in rabbits. *J. Bone Miner. Metab.* 2008;26(1):53-9.

[33] Oestergaard S, Sondergaard BC, Hoegh-Andersen P, Henriksen K, Qvist P, Christiansen C et al. Effects of ovariectomy and estrogen therapy on type II collagen degradation and structural integrity of articular cartilage in rats: implications of the time of initiation. *Arthritis Rheum.* 2006; 54(8): 2441-51.

[34] Morisset S, Patry C, Lora M, Brum-Fernandes AJ. Regulation of cyclooxygenase-2 expression in bovine chondrocytes in culture by interleukin 1alpha, tumor necrosis factor-alpha, glucocorticoids, and 17beta-estradiol. *J. Rheumatol.* 1998;25(6):1146-53.

[35] Claassen H, Schunke M, Kurz B. Estradiol protects cultured articular chondrocytes from oxygen-radical-induced damage. *Cell Tissue Res.* 2005; 319(3): 439-45.

[36] Kou XX, Wu YW, Ding Y, Hao T, Bi RY, Gan YH et al. 17beta-estradiol aggravates temporomandibular joint inflammation through the NF-kappaB pathway in ovariectomized rats. *Arthritis Rheum.* 2011; 63(7): 1888-97.

[37] Nevitt MC, Felson DT, Williams EN, Grady D. The effect of estrogen plus progestin on knee symptoms and related disability in postmenpausal women: The Heart and Estrogen/Progestin Replacement Study, a randomized, double-blind, placebo-controlled trial. *Arthritis Rheum.* 2001;44(4):811-8.

In: Estrogens   ISBN 978-1-62081-747-6
Editors: V. Thompson and A. Watson   © 2012 Nova Science Publishers, Inc.

Chapter 4

ESTROGEN IN REGULATING THE GENDER DISPARITY OF HEPATOCELLULAR CARCINOMA

*Shiou-Hwei Yeh**
Department of Microbiology,
National Taiwan University College of Medicine,
Taipei, Taiwan

ABSTRACT

Hepatocellular carcinoma (HCC) is one of the leading cancers in the world, which is an ultimate outcome of chronic hepatitis with persistent inflammation. Men have a higher incidence of HCC than women. Not only limited to the incidence, this sex difference is also reflected by the clinical course of disease progression and prognosis. The evidence from epidemiologic and animal studies suggested that this gender disparity might be caused by either the stimulatory effects of androgen and/or the protective effects of estrogen. The studies from the N'-N'-diethylnitro-samine (DEN) induced HCC mouse model provided a mechanism for the protective role of estrogen in female HCC. Estrogen was found able to protect hepatocytes from malignant transformation via down-regulation of the secretion of IL-6 from Kupffer cells, a critical process in this

* Correspondence to: Shiou-Hwei Yeh, Ph.D., Associate Professor, Department of Microbiology, National Taiwan University College of Medicine, No. 1, Jen-Ai Road, Section 1, Taipei 100, Taiwan. Fax: 886-2-23825962; E-mail: shyeh@ntu.edu.tw.

mouse model. Moreover, functioning as a strong endogenous antioxidant, estrogen can protect the hepatic steatosis and fibrosis in female livers, which are associated with the increased risk of HCC. It thus raised a unique function of estrogen axis in protecting hepatocarcinogenesis, which is in contrast to its tumor promoting roles in most other female cancers, such as breast cancer and ovarian cancer. Intriguingly, suppression of the ERα protein by overexpression of miR-18a, which occur preferentially in female HCC, was identified as a novel mechanism to block the tumor protective function of estrogen in female HCC. Several critical issues about the estrogen pathway in hepatocarcino-genesis still remained to be clarified, including the detail mechanisms underlying the tumor protective function of estrogen pathway in HCC, the key factor(s) involved in regulating the process, and also its interaction with the hepatitis viruses. Prospectively, the results can help design strategies by targeting to this estrogen axis for preventing or treatment of HCC.

INTRODUCTION

The incidence of hepatocellular carcinoma (HCC) ranks fifth for cancers worldwide and causes about half-a-million deaths every year [1]. HCC is usually an ultimate outcome of chronic hepatitis with persistent inflammation [2-5], caused by hepatitis B virus (HBV) or hepatitis C virus (HCV) infections or by alcoholic/metabolic etiologies [6, 7].

As chronic HBV or HCV infections are causally associated with HCC in more then 80% of HCC [1], the best strategies to prevent HCC are to eradicate the viral infections. Vaccine for HBV has been successfully developed. Vaccination of newborns against HBV has been initiated worldwide and has effectively reduced persistent HBV infections from 15% in the prevaccination era to 1% in the postvaccination era [8].

However, the adults who were infected before the era of universal vaccination are still with high risk for HCC. For example, there still remains more than 350 million HBsAg carriers in the world [1]. Accordingly, the antiviral therapy by nucleos(t)ide analogues (NAs) was developed for efficiently reducing the HBV replication in chronic hepatitis B (CHB) patients, but the process will select drug-resistant mutants in the long run [9].

For hepatitis C, there is no vaccine available now. Although fortunately there is effective therapy that can cure hepatitis C in about 50% of treated patients [6, 10], however the treatment is very expensive and not affordable for the majority of HCV carriers. Therefore, there still remains a large population of patients infected with HBV or HCV at high risk of HCC in their lifetime.

In addition to the major risk factor of hepatitis virus infection, non-viral risk factors also contribute to hepatocarcinogenesis, including alcoholism, aflatoxin exposure, autoimmune hepatitis, and obesity-related fatty liver disease [6, 7]. Notably, although the incidence of HCC in the areas endemic for viral infection is substantially declining, such as eastern Asia and sub-Saharan

Africa for HBV infection and Japan for HCV infection, the incidence increases in the low-rate countries, such as USA and Europe countries [6, 7, 11, 12]. HCC seems to become a new health concern in these highly developed countries. Understanding of the molecular carcinogenic mechanisms and the unique pathogenic biology of HCC and then design the corresponding therapeutic strategies is therefore became an imperative issue worldwide.

Since HCC is well accepted as a consequence of genetic aberrations [13], increasing genome-wide analyses revealed profiles of the genetic changes, the protein coding genes, the miRNA expression patterns, and even the proteomic and the comparative rodent mapping data of HCCs [14]. Integration of these profiles can help classify HCCs into subgroups undergoing distinct carcinogenic pathways.

Accordingly, several major hepatocarcinogenic pathways have been delineated [15-19], including the Wnt signaling pathway, the insulin-like growth factor (IGF] signaling pathway, the Ras/MAPK signaling pathway, and the dysregulation of the G1/S cell cycle transition.

More recently, several other pathways were also implicated in hepatocarcinogenesis, including the mTOR pathway [20], the c-Met pathway [15], the JAK/STAT pathway [21], and the Hedgehog pathway [22]. These pathways might confer hepatocytes with the capabilities of tumor cells, such as invasiveness, limitless replication, or angiogenesis, and allow them to become malignant and metastatic [23].

The specific pathways involved in each subgroup of HCC can help identify the putative targets for designing the cognate molecular-targeted therapies [17]. Based on this rationale, several drugs have been developed targeting to specific carcinogenic pathways, but only one drug, the sorafenib (one multikinase inhibitor against vascular endothelial growth factor receptor, the platelet-derived growth factor receptor, and Raf), has been proven effective and become the first drug approved for treatment of advanced HCCs [17].

However, even the sorafenib can only improve the overall survival of patients with advanced HCC for around 3 months [24]. How to increase the treatment efficacy of HCC, either by identification of new target(s) for anti-tumor therapy or by improving the current targeted therapy strategies, is an imperative issue in this field. Presumably, clear delineation of the causal carcinogenic pathway(s) involved in each HCC can help selection of patients for proper and effective targeted therapy [25, 26]. But until now, this goal is still not achievable due to the great heterogeneity of the carcinogenic pathways involved in HCC. Therefore, there still needs great efforts for exploring the novel and causative hepatocarcinogenic mechanism(s) for the development and application of effective targeted therapies to properly selected patients, maybe in a combination manner.

HCC OCCURS PREFERENTIALLY IN MALES, WITH THE SEX DIFFERENCE STARTING FROM CHRONIC HEPATITIS

In addition to the hepatitis virus infection, alcoholism, aflatoxin exposure, autoimmune hepatitis, and fatty liver disease, male gender is also considered as one major risk factor of HCC [6, 7]. One intriguing universal epidemiologic characteristic of HCC is the prominent male dominance, with the male: female ratio ranging from 1.5-11:1 from different series of analysis [1]. Not only limited to the incidence, this sex difference is also reflected by the poor prognosis and more HCC causing deaths in men than in women [1]. Both the rate for spontaneous survival and survival after resection is better in female HCC [27, 28]. Interestingly, all these advantages for female HCC patients are attenuated after menopause, with increased cirrhotic and HCC cases occurring in older females [29]. The age-specific male to female ratio of HCC cases is thus significantly different between the two groups of patients stratified by the menopausal age (50 years old), with lower proportion of female HCC in the younger group of patients compared with the older group of patients [29].

The effects of gender on clinical features were well documented both for HBV and HCV related liver diseases. Notably, the sex difference occurs in hepatitis B patients starting from the stage of chronic hepatitis [30], suggesting the causative factors actually contributes early in the carcinogenic process. Male sex was identified as a risk factor for the reactivation of hepatitis B in the inactive carriers (positive HBe antibody with normal ALT levels), which confers higher incidence for subsequent cirrhosis and HCC [31, 32]. The same trend was also reported for the asymptomatic HBeAg negative HBV carriers with baseline ALT less than two times the upper limit of normal [33]. Moreover, the results from the long term cohort studies showed the higher percentage of females to achieve seroconversion of HBeAg and HBsAg compared to males [34] [35], which raised hypothesis that females might have more active immune responses against HBV infection than males. Another evidence supporting this hypothesis came from the observation that the chronic HBsAg carrier rate was lower in females then males vaccinated at birth and followed for over 18 years [36]. The involvement of estrogen in regulating the immune response should be an important issue worthy to be extensively explored. For HCV infected patients, male gender is associated with increased rate of fibrosis progression [37]. Male HCV patients are also less responsive to IFN therapy and have higher incidence for early decompensation [37]. The gender effect on hepatocarcinogenesis thus starts relatively early before the HCC occurrence.

Investigating the factors causing such gender disparity in hepato-carcinogenesis has long been considered as a key for unrevealing one critical carcinogenic pathway in HCC. Sex specific differences in exposure to the risk factors were considered as one possible causative factor, for example the male habit for more frequent smoking and alcohol intake. But in addition to the social environment and lifestyle, the epidemiological and experimental evidence further pointed out the sex steroid hormones, both the androgen and estrogen, might function as the major regulatory factors [38]. Since it was noted that the male dominance is more evident in HBV than in HCV related HCC, with the male to female ratio as 3–7:1 for HBV-related HCC and 1.5–3:1 for HCV-related HCC [39, 40], the viral factors are thus also suggested involved in the regulation.

THE INVOLVEMENT OF ANDROGEN AXIS IN PROMOTING MALE HCC

For androgen axis, the male predominance of HCC has implications related to the testosterone and androgen receptor (AR) activities. Human epidemiological studies showed that elevated testosterone levels and the presence of genetic polymorphisms linked to increased androgen activity were significantly associated with the increased risk of HCC in male HBsAg carriers [41, 42]. In rodent HCC models, castration or treatment with anti-androgen agents can protect male rodents from tumor development [43]. Therefore, upregulation of the androgen pathway in male patients is implicated able to accelerate the carcinogenic process.

Recently, the critical involvement of AR pathway in male hepato-carcinogenesis has been well demonstrated in the N'-N'-diethylnitrosamine (DEN) induced HCC mouse model. Specific knock-out of AR expression in hepatocytes delayed the development of DEN induced HCC and also decreased the number of resulting liver tumors, suggesting the active AR pathway in augmenting the HCC risk [44]. Moreover, an intriguing interaction between the specific viral protein of HBV X protein (HBx) and the androgen signaling pathway was recently established, showing that HBx can enhance the transcriptional activity of AR in a ligand concentration-dependent manner, mainly through its effects on the c-Src and GSK-3β kinase pathways [45, 46]. Because of the higher androgen level, the augmentation of the AR pathway is more profound and makes HCC more likely in males. This observation explains the more evident male preference for HBV-related HCC [45]. Because this chapter focuses on the functional role of estrogen axis in hepato-carcinogenesis, the details of the involvement of androgen axis in male hepatocarcinogenesis might need to reference with some other recent review articles [6, 38, 47].

THE INVOLVEMENT OF ESTROGEN AXIS IN PROTECTING FEMALE HCC: EPIDEMIOLOGICAL EVIDENCE AND ANIMAL STUDIES

In addition to the androgen axis, the epidemiological study also suggested the involvement of the estrogen axis in regulating the gender disparity of HCC. But in contrast to the tumor promoting activity of androgen axis, the increased activity of estrogen in females seems to function in a protective manner for hepatocarcinogenesis. The risk of HCC in females was shown to be inversely related to the age at menopause and to the number of full-term pregnancies [48]. In addition, early oophorectomy (at age ≤ 50) was identified as a risk factor for HCC in females, whereas postmenopausal hormone replacement therapy was shown to be a protective factor [48]. This is consistent with animal studies in which ovariectomy increased the susceptibility to HCC in female mice [49, 50]. The role of estrogen axis in hepatocarcinogenesis is thus in contrast with that for other female tumors from the estrogen-responsive tissues, such as the breasts, the uterus, and the ovary. For these female tumors, the estrogen is well characterized to function in a tumor promoter manner [51].

This estrogen mediated contradictory carcinogenic effect has been further supported by the association analyses in the population-based prospective studies by Japan Public Health Center, for the association between the cancer risk and the intake of isoflavone-containing foods. Isofalvones show a similar structure as 17beta-estradiol and have an anti-estrogenic effect in women and estrogenic effect in men.

The results indicated that frequent isoflavone consumption is associated with an increased risk of HCC [52] but in contrast associated with a reduced risk of breast cancer in women [53, 54]. It thus implicated the functional role of estrogen pathway as tumor promoter in breast cancers and as tumor protector in liver cancers in female patients.

Although most of the epidemiologic evidence suggested the tumor protective role of estrogen in female HCC, however some contentions in the literature go against the hypothesis. Long-term use of oral contraceptives was identified as an inducer of female benign hepatomas, including adenoma and FNH [55-57].

Different carcinogenic mechanisms mediated by estrogen pathway were thus implicated for FNH/adenoma and HCC. Actually, distinct profiles of genetic aberrations between HCC and benign FNH/adenoma, revealed by comparative genomic hybridization studies, is in line to support this possibility [58].

The results from animal studies also showed some controversial results about the role of estrogen in hepatocarcinogenesis, either function in a tumor protective or in a tumor promoting manner. In rodent HCC models, ovariectomy was reported able to increase the susceptibility of HCC in female mice [49, 50].

Shimizu *et al.* also demonstrated a suppressive effect of estradiol admini-stration in hepatocarcinogenesis using the DEN, 2-acetylaminofluorene, partial hepatectomy HCC model [59]. In contrast, the synthetic estrogen was found with ability to promote the hepatocarcinogenesis after initiation with DEN treatment [60-62], which in turn will not occur in the absence of the initiation event. It thus raised a possibility that the estrogen might have tumor promoter effect once the tumorigenic process initiates by other carcinogenic factors.

WILD TYPE AND VARIANT ESTROGEN RECEPTORS IN NORMAL AND HCC LIVER TISSUES

Estrogen stimulates a variety of biological activities mainly through two receptors, the ERα and . The ERs are members of the family βER of nuclear receptors and function as transcriptional activators in a ligand dependent manner in most cases [63]. Differential expression of wild type and variant forms of ERs has been reported in normal liver tissues and in HCC. ERα is the major type of ER expressed in the hepatocytes was found elevated in the biliocytes; ER with reactive cholangiocyte proliferation, suggesting its involvement in the proliferative activities of cholangiocytes [64]. Recently, ER was reported to express more often in HCV patients than in HBV patients [65], with its functional role in HCV related liver diseases remained unclear.

By the ligand binding assay, most of the reports showed that the expression of cytosolic or the nuclear ER is decreased in HCC specimens compared to the normal liver tissues [66-68]. Consistently, revealed by IHC staining, both the wild-type ERαexpressed more often in the liver and ER tissues of patients with chronic liver disease compared with those of HCC [69]. However, some contradictory results were also reported that ERs level did not change during carcinogenic process [70, 71]. This might be due to the relatively low expression of ERs in hepatocytes, which limits the detection sensitivity of ERs by IHC staining [47]. To overcome the limitation of IHC staining, Liu *et al.* used the western blot analysis to conclusively evaluate the ERα expression in HCC, showing that ERα protein is decreased in ~60% of HCC compared with the corresponding non-tumorous tissues [72]. This trend fits to the tumor protective role of estrogen pathway in liver tissues, which could be blocked during the carcinogenic process by down regulation of the cognate receptor ERα.

In addition to the wild type ERα, a deletion variant of ERα lacking of exon 5 was frequently identified in HCC, namely vERα [73]. Being lacking of the hormone binding domain, vERα was found to maintain a constitutive transcriptional regulatory activity [74], and not responsive to the estrogen or the anti-estrogen tamoxifen [75, 76]. Notably, vERα occurs preferentially in HBV-infected patients [77], and was identified in male patients with high risk of HCC [75, 76]. Not only associated with the higher clinical aggressiveness, presence of vERα in HCC was found a very strong negative predictor of survival in inoperable HCC patients, which is even worse in the HBsAg-positive patients [78, 79]. Intriguingly, when compared with the commonly applied Okuda and CLIP clinical scoring systems, the ER classification of HCC by evaluation of the presence of wild-type or variant ER transcripts in HCC is considered a even more powerful molecular scoring system for predicting of survival in HCC patients [75].

Regarding to the functional role of vERα in liver pathophysiology, Farinati *et al.* found that the presence of vERα in liver was associated with higher level of DNA damage induced by oxidative stress [80]. In addition, in the cell culture system, Han *et al.* demonstrated that vERα can interact with wild type ERα and functions as a dominant negative receptor for wild type ERα, to repress the ligand stimulate ERα transcriptional activity [81]. This seems to be contradictory to the previous observation about vERα as a constitutive active form of ERα to activate the transcription in a ligand independent manner. The biological significance of this observation for *in vivo* hepatocarcinogenesis warrants further clarification.

MOLECULAR MECHANISMS FOR THE PROTECTIVE ROLE OF ESTROGEN AXIS IN FEMALE HCC

Because the epidemiological evidence strongly suggested the role of estrogen axis in protecting the female HCC, understating the underlying molecular mechanism(s) become important for the development of matching anti-tumor strategy. This includes [1] how the estrogen axis implements its tumor protective effect, and also [2] what is the key regulatory mechanism(s) for the down-regulation of the activity of estrogen axis in the carcinogenic process. Increasing studies focused on both critical issues and several novel mechanisms have been disclosed recently.

As mentioned above in the introduction, the persistent chronic inflamemation process predisposes to HCC irrespective of the etiologies. Since the sex disparity occurs from the stage of chronic hepatitis, we expect this axis might have its anti-tumor function starting from this early stage, to against the inflammation process. During liver inflammation, the immune-related cells and the inflammatory factors they produce are enriched in the local inflamematory microenvironment and function as the major regulators mediating the inflammation process. The macrophages (Kupffer cells), T cells, and other immune cells are recruited to the microenvironment and release the proinflammatory factors, including the cytokines (such as TNF-α, IL-1β, IL-6, etc.) and chemokines (such as CXCL8, CXCR4, etc.) [2, 82-85].

An interaction between the inflammatory cells and the hepatocytes occurs within this microenvironment. The protumorigenic factors released by the immune cells can target and activate several transcriptional activators within the hepatocytes, including NF-κB, signal transducer and activator of transcription 3 (STAT3), hypoxia-inducible factor 1α (HIF-1α), and so on [82]. Activation of these transcription factors not only can increase the tumorigenic activity of hepatocytes but also can lead to the production of some more inflammatory mediators, which further recruit and activate immune cells in the liver tissues [2, 82-85].

Such an amplification loop establishes a cancer-prone inflammatory microenvironment and predisposes the subsequent HCC formation.

Notably, NF-κB was identified as the critical factor in regulating the interplay between target hepatocytes and immune cells in favor of tumorigenic processes [85, 86], with the evidence mainly derived from the DEN induced mouse HCC model.

In this model, IL-1α released from DEN damaged necrotic hepatocytes can initiate the induction and release of IL-6 from Kupffer cells, mainly through the activation of NF-κB pathway [87]. Release of IL-6 from Kupffer cells can then regulate the NF-κB activity in the hepatocytes, which was identified to be critical for the subsequent hepatocarcinogenesis in this tumor model [88, 89].

Intriguingly, the gender disparity of HCC occurrence is also found in this DEN-induced HCC mouse model, with the tumor incidence higher in male than female mice [89]. Both orchidectomy and implantation the estrogen tablets in male mice can decrease the tumor incidence. In contrast, ovary-ectomy and / or testosterone supplement for the female mice can signify-cantly increase the occurrence of HCC [50].

Therefore, both the androgen and estrogen axis were implicated in determining the gender disparity of HCC in this model. Prof. Karin and his colleagues first noted that administration of DEN can induce higher serum IL-6 in male than in female mice, which can be abrogated by the administration of 17β-estroadiol (E2) to the male mice [90]. Ovariectomy of female mice could increase the serum IL-6, and which could be prevented by E2 administration.

The results suggested that estrogen axis is critical for the maintaining the lower level of serum IL-6 in females. To evaluate if the sex difference of IL-6 release accounts for the gender disparity of HCC development, they examined the DEN-induced HCC in IL-6 knockout IL-6$^{-/-}$ mice. The gender differences in hepatocarcinogenesis, including the tumor incidence and survival rate, were abolished in the IL-6$^{-/-}$ mice, suggesting that estrogen mediated down-regulation of IL-6 is critical for the gender disparity of HCC in this tumor model [90]. Since the IL-6 is mainly released from the Kupffer cells in liver, they have focused on the Kupffer cells to further delineate the mechanism underlying the estrogen in regulating the IL-6 secretion. Aided by the knockout mice, ERα was identified responsible for the protective effect of estrogen in the Kupffer cells. Moreover, the Toll-like receptor (TLR) adaptor protein MyD88 was found critical for the DEN-induced release of IL-6 from Kupffer cells. Through ERα, estrogen can inhibit the promoter activity of IL-6 through decreasing the MyD88 mediated activation of NF-κB. This prevents the IL-6 inducing tumorigenic effect on hepatocytes, mainly through activation of STAT3 and persistence of the JNK kinase activity in hepatocytes [90]. Therefore, the results from this mouse model well demonstrated that estrogen could protect hepatocytes from malignant transformation via down-regulation of the secretion of IL-6 from Kupffer cells, a critical process in the DEN-induced HCC (Figure 7.1).

The results from mouse model provided a mechanism for the protective role of estrogen against HCC in females, which could occur at the stage of chronic hepatitis. Actually, this is also supported by the human studies. For females, decline in ovarian function with menopause is usually associated with spontaneous increases in proinflammatory cytokines, including IL-6, TNF-α, and IL-1β [91], which associates with the persistent liver injury. Supplement with estrodiol for the postmenopausal women can effectively decrease the spontaneous production of IL-6 by peripheral blood mononuclear cells [92]. Therefore, estroadiol has a hepatoprotective effect against persistent inflammation by inhibiting proinflammatory cytokine production was well illustrated.

THE MECHANISMS OF ESTROGEN AXIS IN PREVENTING HEPATIC FIBROSIS AND STEATOSIS

In addition to HCC, estrogen axis was also reported to be associated with some other hepatocarcinogenesis related liver diseases, including the hepatic fibrosis and the hepatic steatosis. Hepatic fibrosis, which is caused by collagen deposition, is a consequence of severe liver damage that usually occurs in patients with chronic liver disease. The collagens are produced by the hepatic stellate cells (HSCs). HSCs are the primary target cells for inflammatory and peroxidative stimuli in the injured liver [93], mainly activated by the reactive oxygen species (ROS) derived from the lipid peroxidative processes in hepatocytes [94]. Estrogen was reported as a strong endogenous antioxidant that can reduce the lipid peroxide levels in the liver tissues [80, 95].

This could be mediated through various regulatory mechanisms, including suppressing of the ROS generation and lipid peroxidation, suppressing the antioxidant protective systems of the superoxide dismutase and glutathione B (the peroxidase, activation of AP-1 and NF- redox sensitive transcription factors), and up-regulating the Bcl-2 (a suppressor of lipid peroxidation) [96, 97].

In this regard, estrogen can thus block the activation of HSCs, the subsequent collagen synthesis, and the resulting hepatofiborgenesis.

Meanwhile, estrogen could protect the hepatocytes from oxidative stress induced DNA damage and genetic alterations, which generally lead to the HCC through a multistep process.

The evidence from both animal and human studies well supported the protective role of estrogen in hepatic fibrosis. In the hepatic fibrosis model of rats, the hepatic fibrosis could be effectively suppressed by the administration of estrogen [98-100].

For human studies, male gender and older age (>50 years) are associated with a more rapid progression of hepatic fibrosis [101], and also are predictors for cirrhosis in patients with chronic HBV infections [102, 103].

In addition to the hepatic fibrosis, the hepatic steatosis is also frequently identified in the liver diseases, in around 30~50% of chronic hepatitis B and 30~70% of chronic hepatitis C [104, 105]. The high percentage of hepatic steatosis in hepatitis livers suggested a direct cytopathic effect by hepatitis viral factors.

This has been supported by the transgenic mouse either expressing HCV core protein or HBV X protein, showing progressive hepatic steatosis predisposing the occurrence of HCC [106-108]. Hepatic steatosis is cause by the deposition of triglycerides via the accumulation of free fatty acids in hepatocytes. During chronic hepatitis, impaired oxidation of the accumulated fatty acids causes the accumulation of lipid peroxidation products, which further leads to the activation of HSCs and the subsequent hepatic fibrosis.

In the process, the estrogen axis seems to also play a protective role for preventing the hepatic steatosis. First, it was noted that the tamoxifen (an antiestrogen compound) treatment was associated with an increased risk of fatty liver [109, 110]. Moreover, in the aromatase-deficient mouse model (lack of estrogen production), Nemoto *et al.* found hepatic steatosis occurred spontaneously, through impaired gene expression and enzyme activities of fatty acid -oxidation [111].

The hepatic steatosis in this model can be recovered by estradiol replacement, suggesting the pivotal role of estrogen in maintaining hepatic lipid homeostasis. This also explains the greater progression of liver injury with steatosis in male patients [112]. Therefore, the estrogen axis also protects these two HCC prone liver diseases of hepatic fibrosis and steatosis through distinct molecular mechanisms.

The Regulatory Mechanisms for the Down-Regulation of ERα in Female HCC

In addition to have tumor protective effect on Kuppfer cells, the possibility that the estrogen axis also have tumor protective effect for the hepatocytes is highly suggested.

This is mainly due to the findings from clinical specimens, showing ERα protein (the major estrogen receptor mediating the function of estrogen in liver tissues) to be significantly decreased in the HCC tissues [69]. Not only revealed by the receptor binding assay and the IHC staining (detectable only in 15-40% of female HCCs) [27, 113, 114], this trend has been further conclusively supported by Western blot analysis (down-regulated in ~60% of female HCCs) [72]. However, the contribution of ERα decrease in hepatocytes for the female carcinogenesis and also the underlying molecular mechanism(s) is not well disclosed yet, although its effect for decreasing the proliferation activity of hepatoma cell lines has been well demonstrated [72].

Recently, several reports tried to address the critical issue about how is ERα protein decreased in female HCC, as a mechanism for blocking its tumor protective effect in hepatocytes.

Shen et al. documented a mechanism for ER□ downregulation in HCC by the methylation of a CpG island at the promoter region of ER□ [115]. However, decrease of ER□RNA in HCC was not found in female HCC by different series of studies [65, 69, 77, 116]. Moreover, Liu et al. showed that most HCC with decreased ER□ protein did not show the decreased RNA of ER□, making this mechanism not a major regulatory mechanism contributing to the decrease of ER□protein in female HCC.

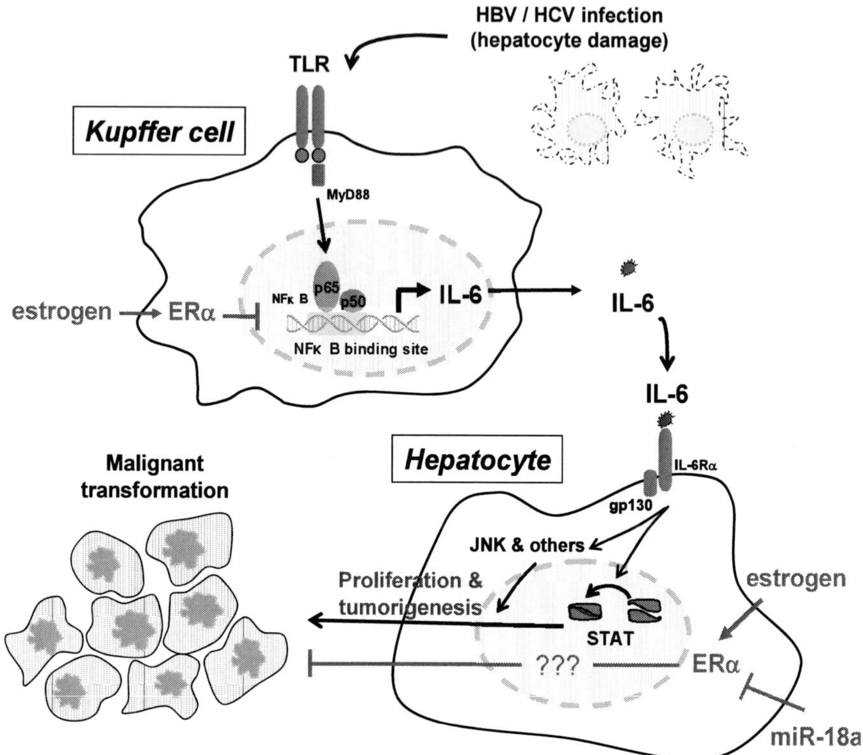

Figure 1. The tumor protective effect of estrogen in hepatocarcinogenesis, both targeting to Kuppfer cells and the hepatocytes, respectively. The immune cells are recruited to the liver due to the virus infection and/or liver damages, including macrophages (Kupffer cells), T cells, and others. Among them, the Kupffer cells could be activated through TLR-MyD88-NF-κB pathway to release the IL-6, which in turn stimulates the proliferation and transformation of hepatocytes by binding to the cognate receptors on hepatocytes. Estrogen has its anti-tumor effect by suppressing the release of IL-6, mediated through the ERα receptor to block the activation of NF-κB in the Kupffer cells. In addition, estrogen can also have its anti-tumor effect on the hepatocytes, with the underlying mechanism remained to be clarified. This anti-tumor effect could be suppressed in female HCC by the elevation of miR-18a, which targets and suppresses the expression of ERα in hepatocytes.

Intriguingly, our recent study has revealed one novel microRNA regulatory mechanism for the decreased ERα protein in female HCC. By comparing the expression pattern of miRNAs between male and female HCCs, one specific miRNA, miR-18a, was identified to be preferentially increased in female HCCs [72]. This sex difference of miR-18a expression pattern was not identified in FNHs and adenomas, suggesting it as a mechanism specific for HCC. The gene *ESR1*, which encodes the estrogen receptor-α (ERα), was predicted as a target for miR-18a, by PicTar and TargetScan algorithms [117, 118]. In line to support this, increased levels of miR-18a in HCC tissues were noted to be well correlated with the reduced ERα expression. Further molecular evidence demonstrated that miR-18a can regulate ERα protein expression by binding to its putative 3′UTR target sites. It regulates the ERα protein mainly at the posttranscriptional level, since only little effect on the mRNA level of ERα was observed for the overexpression of miR-18a. To further identify the step(s) deregulated during the biogenesis of miR-18a which lead to the increased miR-18a in female HCCs, the correlation between the level of miR-18a and its precursor molecules, the pri-miR-18a and pre-miR-18a, were compared. No significant correlation between pri- and miR-18a was identified, in contrast a significant correlation between pre- and miR-18a has been identified. The elevation of mature miR-18a was thus possibly caused by a deregulated processing of pri-miR-18a to pre-miR-18a. The detail mechanisms and the RNA-binding proteins involved in accelerating the processing of miR-18a in female HCC await further investigation. This study thus provides a novel miRNA-mediated regulatory mechanism for controlling ERα expression in hepatocytes, which attributes to the decreased activity of estrogen axis in female hepatocarcinogenesis (Figure 1).

THE INTERACTION BETWEEN THE HEPATITIS VIRUS B AND ESTROGEN PATHWAY

As the virus-related hepatocarcinogenesis is an interplay between the hepatitis viruses and the hepatocytes, both viral and host genomes contribute to the final pathogenic outcome. Therefore, not only the host factors but also the viral factors might involve in the regulation of gender disparity of HCC. This has already been well demonstrated in the case of HBV. The results from our previous study showed that HBx can enhance the transcriptional activity of AR to enhance the carcinogenic effect of androgen axis in males [45, 46]. Our recent study further identified that the androgen pathway can enhance the RNA transcription of HBV in a ligand dependent manner. This is mediated through the targeting of ligand stimulated AR to the androgen responsive elements in enhancer I region of HBV genome. Such a positive feedback loop between AR activation and HBV transcription can potentiate the hepato-carcinogenesis by persisting the activation of the AR carcinogenic pathway in HBV infected males.

Intriguingly, in contrast to the effect of androgen pathway to increase the HBV mRNA synthesis, Almog *et al.* reported that estrogen can decrease the HBV mRNA level [119]. By implantation of HepG 2.2.15 cells into the athymic mice, they found that the derived tumors collected from the male mice showed higher HBV mRNA than that collected from female mice.

Treatment of male mice with estrogen can significantly decrease the HBV mRNA levels, suggesting the suppressive effect of estrogen in the synthesis of HBV mRNA [119]. Apparently, estrogen and androgen pathways have opposite effects on HBV mRNA transcription. This is consistent with their opposite roles in hepatocarcinogenesis, but for regulating the HBV life cycle in addition to affect the host factors.

Moreover, Han *et al.* demonstrated that HBx can inhibit the transcriptional activity of ERα [81]. HBx interacts with ERα, which in turn recruits the histone deacetylases 1 (HDAC1) to the estrogen responsive element in the promoter region of cellular target genes and repress the ERα-dependent transcriptional activity [81].

The HBx viral protein thus seems to target and decrease the estrogen pathway to have its tumor promoting activity in female HBV patients. A negative feedback loop thus exists between these two events of [1] HBx inhibits the estrogen activity and [2] estrogen suppresses the HBV transcription, which can decrease the tumor protective activity of estrogen pathway in female HBV patients.

In conclusion, the interactive effect between HBV and the sex steroid hormones seems to be contradictory between the androgen and estrogen pathways. For HCV, currently there is lack of information about the cross talk between estrogen pathway and the HCV viral factors and is worthy to be extensively investigated.

CONCLUSION

According to the epidemiological and also the experimental studies, both androgen and estrogen sex steroids could attribute to the gender disparity of HCC, but with distinct roles in each gender. The higher activity of androgen pathway functions as a tumor-promoting factor in male hepatocarcinogenesis, and the higher activity of the estrogen pathway functions as a tumor-suppressing factor in female hepatocarcinogenesis. As both mechanisms function in a ligand-dependent manner, both the ligand and the receptor of these sex hormones are suggested to be included in assessing the relative risk of HCC patients of each gender. Moreover, the evidence from epidemiological and preclinical studies has suggested the androgen and estrogen axes as potential targets for targeted therapy. Several clinical trials have tested the efficacy of hormonal treatment in HCC patients, both targeting to the androgen and estrogen axes [120].

To focus on the estrogen pathway, the anti-estrogen tamoxifen has been developed and proven very effective for the patients with hormone-sensitive breast cancer. Tamoxifen inhibits the activity of estrogen by competitive antagonism of the receptor sites. Therefore, the level of estrogen receptor expression are the best predictor of benefit from tamoxifen [121]. However, application of the same criteria to HCC remains some problems. IHC staining is relatively low, First, the percentage of HCC with positive ER which is even more complicated by the great variability protein levels and also by the α of the ER (exon 5 deleted) in the positive cases [76, presence of the variant form of ER 79]. Secondly, from the viewpoint of the tumor protective role signaling pathway of ER in female HCC, block of estrogen pathway by tamoxifen could have tumor promoting rather than tumor preventing effect in female HCC. Under such presumption, we might not expect the effective therapeutic effect of the targeted therapy by blocking the estrogen pathway, at least for the female ones. These two issues will be included for later discussion about the results obtained from tamoxifen trails for HCC patients.

In the last decades, a number of randomized controlled trials have tested the efficacy of tamoxifen for patients with HCC, but coming out rather conflicting results [120, 122-125]. The results from the earlier small-randomized trials showed marginal increase in overall survival with the use of tamoxifen in advanced HCC [122, 123], which calls for a larger randomized controlled trial to definitely evaluate the efficacy of tamoxifen treatment. However, it was disappointing that a subsequent larger randomized study by CLIP did not show overall survival advantage by the administration of tamoxifen [126]. Due to the great variations protein expression levels and the α of the ER in HCCs, one hypothesis presence of deletion variant of ER has been raised that proper selection of the status could improve the efficacy of tamoxifenαHCC cases according to the ER status could include both the expression level and the treatment. The ERα in HCC. Because of the lack of ligand presence or absence of the vER binding region is resistant to the α, vER tamoxifen treatment. Therefore, it is expected that the HCCs containing wild type will be more rather than the vER ERα responsive to the tamoxifen treatment. Actually, the preliminary study for testing this possibility obtained exciting results, showing that the tumor was volume in patients with wild-type ER significantly reduced after tamoxifen treatment [78]. Although still quite preliminary, the possibility that tamoxifen treatment could be effective only in a selected subgroup of patients with HCC is worthy to be studied in the future.

In addition to the status of ERα in HCC some other factors such as the gender factor, might also need to be included for consideration in selecting the patients suitable for tamoxifen treatment. Presumably, a more comprehensive understanding of the molecular mechanisms underlying estrogen pathway in hepatocarcinogenesis is required for identifying such determining factors. For examples, although the tumor protective role of estrogen in female HCC has been well documented, the functional role of this pathway in male HCC remains inconclusive. Clarification of the functional role of wild type in male and deletion variant vERαER hepatocarcinogenesis is critical for determining if male HCC patients (with are more favorable for tamoxifen treatment than female patients. wild type ERα This hypothesis is suggested by the results from animal studies, showing the estrogen pathway to function as tumor promoter in male mice once the tumor initiation events occur [60, 62, 127, 128]. It would be interesting to investigate if this also occurs in human male HCC cases, with the virus infection or some other factors as the initiation events.

Another intriguing issue remains to be clarified is about why the estrogen pathway plays contradictory role in the carcinogenesis of female HCC and other female tumors, such as breast cancers and ovarian cancers. The tissue specific cellular context and also the associated molecular mechanism determining such distinct roles need to be addressed. This will be extremely important since the administration of estrogen to prevent female HCC might at the same time increase the risk for other female tumors due to its tumor promoting role for these tumors. If the key cellular regulator(s) controlling the protective effect of estrogen in hepatocytes can be delineated, the targeted therapy can be designed for the key cellular factor(s) instead of treating the patients with estrogen agonist(s). Hopefully, the goal for preventing HCC but not stimulating the risk of breast cancers could be achieved.

In addition to regulate the cellular carcinogenic mechanisms, the effect of estrogen pathway to interact with the hepatitis viruses at the stage of chronic hepatitis is another important issue with clinical implication. For example, it was reported that the estrogen pathway can block the transcription of HBV, as a mechanism for explaining the higher viral titer found in male HBV patients [119]. Although the detail mechanism remained to be clarified, it raised a possibility that estrogen could be used to block the virus replication as an anti-viral drug, especially for the male patients. Again, survey of the detail mechanisms can help identify the key cellular factors as the alternative targets for designing safer treatment, instead of applying the estrogen which might increase the risk of other female tumors. Secondly, the finding that females are easier to get seroconversion of HBeAg and HBsAg than males [34, 35] suggested the function of estrogen pathway in stimulating higher immune surveillance activity. The mechanism for estrogen in regulating the immune clearance activity in patients infected with hepatitis viruses is an intriguing issue to be studied. Actually, the male vulnerability is evidently identified in most infectious diseases, implicating this mechanism could be applied to explain of the sex difference of other infectious diseases.

To focus on the mechanism regulating the decreased activity of estrogen pathway in female HCC, down-regulation through elevation of miR-18a has been of ERα identified preferentially in the female HCC [72]. How does miR-18a elevate during the carcinogenic process is the next question to be addressed. Since miR-18a miRNA is expressed as part of a cluster of intronic RNAs of miR-17–92 [129]. The mechanism regulating the processing of this specific miRNA within this cluster warrants further investigation. Presumably, targeted to reverse the elevation of the miR-18a in female HCC could restore the anti-tumor activity of estrogen in female HCC, as a potential strategy to against the hepatocarcinogenesis in female patients. In summary, concerning to the estrogen axis as a tumor protector for female hepatocarcinogenesis, through affecting both the host and viral factors, the feasibility to prevent or treat HCC by estrogen administration is worthy to be evaluated.

To avoid the increased risk for other female tumors, further studies will focus on investigation of the detail mechanisms regulating the process. In the long run, some other cellular targets can be identified for designing effective but safer treatment. Moreover, the applicability of such treatment to the male HCC, the major population suffering from high risk of HCC, is also an imperative issue to be examined.

ACKNOWLEDGMENTS

This chapter was supported by National Research Program of Genomic Medicine, National Science Council, Taiwan (NSC97-3112-B-002-030-) and also by National Health Research Institutes, Taiwan (NHRI-EX98-9832BI).

REFERENCES

[1] Parkin, DM; Bray, F; Ferlay, J; Pisani, P. Estimating the world cancer burden: Globocan 2000. *Int. J. Cancer,* 2001 94, 153-156.

[2] Gao, B; Jeong, WI; Tian, Z. Liver: An organ with predominant innate immunity. *Hepatology,* 2008 47, 729-736.

[3] Seitz, HK; Stickel, F. Molecular mechanisms of alcohol-mediated carcinogenesis. *Nat. Rev. Cancer,* 2007 7, 599-612.

[4] Maher, JJ; Leon, P; Ryan, JC. Beyond insulin resistance: Innate immunity in nonalcoholic steatohepatitis. *Hepatology,* 2008 48, 670-678.

[5] Shoelson, SE; Herrero, L; Naaz, A. Obesity, inflammation, and insulin resistance. *Gastroenterology,* 2007 132, 2169-2180.

[6] Tan, A; Yeh, SH; Liu, CJ; Cheung, C; Chen, PJ. Viral heapto-carcinogenesis: from infection to cancer. *Liver Int,* 2008 28, 175-188.

[7] Gomaa, AI; Khan, SA; Toledano, MB; Waked, I; Taylor-Robinson, SD. Hepatocellular carcinoma: epidemiology, risk factors and pathogenesis. *World J. Gastroenterol.,* 2008 14, 4300-4308.

[8] Kao, JH; Chen, DS. Global control of hepatitis B virus infection. *Lancet Infect. Dis.,* 2002 2, 395-403.

[9] Feld, J; Locarnini, S. Antiviral therapy for hepatitis B virus infections: new targets and technical challenges. *J. Clin. Virol.,* 2002 25, 267-283.

[10] Jensen, DM; Ascione, A. Future directions in therapy for chronic hepatitis C. *Antivir. Ther.* 2008 13 Suppl 1, 31-36.

[11] El-Serag, HB; Davila, JA; Petersen, NJ; McGlynn, KA. The continuing increase in the incidence of hepatocellular carcinoma in the United States: an update. *Ann. Intern. Med.,* 2003 139, 817-823.

[12] Deuffic, S; Poynard, T; Buffat, L; Valleron, AJ. Trends in primary liver cancer. *Lancet,* 1998 351, 214-215.

[13] Chen, PJ; Chen, DS. Hepatitis B virus infection and hepatocellular carcinoma: molecular genetics and clinical perspectives. *Semin. Liver Dis.,* 1999 19, 253-262.

[14] Su, WH; Chao, CC; Yeh, SH; Chen, DS; Chen, PJ; Jou, YS. Onco DB.HCC: an integrated oncogenomic database of hepatocellular carcinoma revealed aberrant cancer target genes and loci. *Nucleic. Acids Res.,* 2007 35, D727-731.

[15] Villanueva, A; Newell, P; Chiang, DY; Friedman, SL; Llovet, JM. Genomics and signaling pathways in hepatocellular carcinoma. *Semin. Liver Dis.*, 2007 27, 55-76.

[16] Aravalli, RN; Steer, CJ; Cressman, EN. Molecular mechanisms of hepatocellular carcinoma. *Hepatology,* 2008 48, 2047-2063.

[17] Llovet, JM; Bruix, J. Molecular targeted therapies in hepatocellular carcinoma. *Hepatology,* 2008 48, 1312-1327.

[18] Malumbres, M; Barbacid, M. To cycle or not to cycle: a critical decision in cancer. *Nat Rev Cancer,* 2001 1, 222-231.

[19] Tannapfel, A; Busse, C; Weinans, L; Benicke, M; Katalinic, A; Geissler, F; Hauss, J; Wittekind, C. INK4a-ARF alterations and p53 mutations in hepatocellular carcinomas. *Oncogene,* 2001 20, 7104-7109.

[20] Villanueva, A; Chiang, DY; Newell, P; Peix, J; Thung, S; Alsinet, C; Tovar, V; Roayaie, S; Minguez, B; Sole, M; Battiston, C; van Laarhoven, S; Fiel, MI; Feo, AD; Hoshida, Y; Yea, S; Toffanin, S; Ramos, A; Martignetti, JA; Mazzaferro, V; Bruix, J; Waxman, S; Schwartz, M; Meyerson, M; Friedman, SL; Llovet, JM. Pivotal Role of mTOR Signaling in Hepatocellular Carcinoma. *Gastroenterology,* 2008 135, 1972-1983.

[21] Calvisi, DF; Ladu, S; Gorden, A; Farina, M; Conner, EA; Lee, JS; Factor, VM; Thorgeirsson, SS. Ubiquitous activation of Ras and Jak/Stat pathways in human HCC. *Gastroenterology,* 2006 130, 1117-1128.

[22] Osipo, C; Miele, L. Hedgehog signaling in hepatocellular carcinoma: novel therapeutic strategy targeting hedgehog signaling in HCC. *Cancer Biol. Ther.* 2006 5, 238-239.

[23] Hanahan, D; Weinberg, RA. The hallmarks of cancer. *Cell,* 2000 100, 57-70.

[24] Llovet, JM; Ricci, S; Mazzaferro, V; Hilgard, P; Gane, E; Blanc, JF; de Oliveira, AC; Santoro, A; Raoul, JL; Forner, A; Schwartz, M; Porta, C; Zeuzem, S; Bolondi, L; Greten, TF; Galle, PR; Seitz, JF; Borbath, I; Haussinger, D; Giannaris, T; Shan, M; Moscovici, M; Voliotis, D; Bruix, J. Sorafenib in advanced hepatocellular carcinoma. *N. Engl. J. Med.,* 2008 359, 378-390.

[25] Tome, ME; Johnson, DB; Rimsza, LM; Roberts, RA; Grogan, TM; Miller, TP; Oberley, LW; Briehl, MM. A redox signature score identifies diffuse large B-cell lymphoma patients with a poor prognosis. *Blood,* 2005 106, 3594-3601.

[26] Boyault, S; Rickman, DS; de Reynies, A; Balabaud, C; Rebouissou, S; Jeannot, E; Herault, A; Saric, J; Belghiti, J; Franco, D; Bioulac-Sage, P; Laurent-Puig, P; Zucman-Rossi, J. Transcriptome classification of HCC is related to gene alterations and to new therapeutic targets. *Hepatology,* 2007 45, 42-52.

[27] Ng, IO; Ng, M; Fan, ST. Better survival in women with resected hepatocellular carcinoma is not related to tumor proliferation or expression of hormone receptors. *Am. J. Gastroenterol.,* 1997 92, 1355-1358.

[28] Fukuda, S; Itamoto, T; Amano, H; Kohashi, T; Ohdan, H; Tashiro, H; Asahara, T. Clinicopathologic features of hepatocellular carcinoma patients with compensated cirrhosis surviving more than 10 years after curative hepatectomy. *World J. Surg.* 2007 31, 345-352.

[29] Shimizu, I; Ito, S. Protection of estrogens against the progression of chronic liver disease. *Hepatol. Res.,* 2007 37, 239-247.

[30] Chu, CM; Liaw, YF; Sheen, IS; Lin, DY; Huang, MJ. Sex difference in chronic hepatitis B virus infection: an appraisal based on the status of hepatitis B e antigen and antibody. *Hepatology,* 1983 3, 947-950.

[31] Chu, CM; Liaw, YF. Predictive factors for reactivation of hepatitis B following hepatitis B e antigen seroconversion in chronic hepatitis B. *Gastroenterology,* 2007 133, 1458-1465.

[32] Chu, CM; Liaw, YF. Incidence and risk factors of progression to cirrhosis in inactive carriers of hepatitis B virus. *Am. J. Gastroenterol.,* 2009 104, 1693-1699.

[33] Tai, DI; Lin, SM; Sheen, IS; Chu, CM; Lin, DY; Liaw, YF. Long-term outcome of hepatitis B e antigen-negative hepatitis B surface antigen carriers in relation to changes of alanine aminotransferase levels over time. *Hepatology,* 2009 49, 1859-1867.

[34] Alward, WL; McMahon, BJ; Hall, DB; Heyward, WL; Francis, DP; Bender, TR. The long-term serological course of asymptomatic hepatitis B virus carriers and the development of primary hepatocellular carcinoma. *J. Infect. Dis.,* 1985 151, 604-609.

[35] Zacharakis, GH; Koskinas, J; Kotsiou, S; Papoutselis, M; Tzara, F; Vafeiadis, N; Archimandritis, AJ; Papoutselis, K. Natural history of chronic HBV infection: a cohort study with up to 12 years follow-up in North Greece (part of the Interreg I-II/EC-project). *J. Med. Virol.,* 2005 77, 173-179.

[36] Su, FH; Chen, JD; Cheng, SH; Lin, CH; Liu, YH; Chu, FY. Seroprevalence of Hepatitis-B infection amongst Taiwanese university students 18 years following the commencement of a national Hepatitis-B vaccination program. *J. Med. Virol.,* 2007 79, 138-143.

[37] Poynard, T; Bedossa, P; Opolon, P. Natural history of liver fibrosis progression in patients with chronic hepatitis C. The OBSVIRC, METAVIR, CLINIVIR, and DOSVIRC groups. *Lancet,* 1997 349, 825-832.

[38] De Maria, N; Manno, M; Villa, E. Sex hormones and liver cancer. *Mol. Cell Endocrinol.* 2002 193, 59-63.

[39] Lee, CM; Lu, SN; Changchien, CS; Yeh, CT; Hsu, TT; Tang, JH; Wang, JH; Lin, DY; Chen, CL; Chen, WJ. Age, gender, and local geographic variations of viral etiology of hepatocellular carcinoma in a hyperendemic area for hepatitis B virus infection. *Cancer,* 1999 86, 1143-1150.

[40] Shiratori, Y; Shiina, S; Imamura, M; Kato, N; Kanai, F; Okudaira, T; Teratani, T; Tohgo, G; Toda, N; Ohashi, M. Characteristic difference of hepatocellular carcinoma between hepatitis B- and C- viral infection in Japan. *Hepatology,* 1995 22, 1027-1033.

[41] Yu, MW; Yang, YC; Yang, SY; Cheng, SW; Liaw, YF; Lin, SM; Chen, CJ. Hormonal markers and hepatitis B virus-related hepatocellular carcinoma risk: a nested case-control study among men. *J. Natl. Cancer Inst.,* 2001 93, 1644-1651.

[42] Yu, MW; Cheng, SW; Lin, MW; Yang, SY; Liaw, YF; Chang, HC; Hsiao, TJ; Lin, SM; Lee, SD; Chen, PJ; Liu, CJ; Chen, CJ. Androgen-receptor gene CAG repeats, plasma testosterone levels, and risk of hepatitis B-related hepatocellular carcinoma. *J. Natl. Cancer Inst.,* 2000 92, 2023-2028.

[43] Toh, YC. Effect of neonatal castration on liver tumor induction by N-2-fluorenylacetamide in suckling BALB/c mice. *Carcinogenesis,* 1981 2, 1219-1221.

[44] Ma, WL; Hsu, CL; Wu, MH; Wu, CT; Wu, CC; Lai, JJ; Jou, YS; Chen, CW; Yeh, S; Chang, C. Androgen receptor is a new potential therapeutic target for the treatment of hepatocellular carcinoma. *Gastroenterology,* 2008 135, 947-955, 955.e1-5.

[45] Chiu, CM; Yeh, SH; Chen, PJ; Kuo, TJ; Chang, CJ; Chen, PJ; Yang, WJ; Chen, DS. Hepatitis B virus X protein enhances androgen receptor-responsive gene expression depending on androgen level. *Proc. Natl. Acad. Sci. USA,* 2007 104, 2571-2578.

[46] Yang, WJ; Chang, CJ; Yeh, SH; Lin, WH; Wang, SH; Tsai, TF; Chen, DS; Chen, PJ. Hepatitis B virus X protein enhances the transcriptional activity of the androgen receptor through c-Src and glycogen synthase kinase-3beta kinase pathways. *Hepatology,* 2009 49, 1515-1524.

[47] Kalra, M; Mayes, J; Assefa, S; Kaul, AK; Kaul, R. Role of sex steroid receptors in pathobiology of hepatocellular carcinoma. *World J. Gastroenterol.,* 2008 14, 5945-5961.

[48] Yu, MW; Chang, HC; Chang, SC; Liaw, YF; Lin, SM; Liu, CJ; Lee, SD; Lin, CL; Chen, PJ; Lin, SC; Chen, CJ. Role of reproductive factors in hepatocellular carcinoma: Impact on hepatitis B- and C-related risk. *Hepatology,* 2003 38, 1393-1400.

[49] Vesselinovitch, SD; Itze, L; Mihailovich, N; Rao, KV. Modifying role of partial hepatectomy and gonadectomy in ethylnitrosourea-induced hepatocarcinogenesis. *Cancer Res.,* 1980 40, 1538-1542.

[50] Nakatani, T; Roy, G; Fujimoto, N; Asahara, T; Ito, A. Sex hormone dependency of diethylnitrosamine-induced liver tumors in mice and chemoprevention by leuprorelin. *Jpn J. Cancer Res.,* 2001 92, 249-256.

[51] Pike, MC; Spicer, DV. Hormonal contraception and chemoprevention of female cancers. *Endocr. Relat. Cancer,* 2000 7, 73-83.

[52] Kurahashi, N; Inoue, M; Iwasaki, M; Tanaka, Y; Mizokami, M; Tsugane, S. Isoflavone consumption and subsequent risk of hepato-cellular carcinoma in a population-based prospective cohort of Japanese men and women. *Int. J. Cancer,* 2009 124, 1644-1649.

[53] Yamamoto, S; Sobue, T; Kobayashi, M; Sasaki, S; Tsugane, S. Soy, isoflavones, and breast cancer risk in Japan. *J. Natl. Cancer Inst.,* 2003 95, 906-913.

[54] Iwasaki, M; Inoue, M; Otani, T; Sasazuki, S; Kurahashi, N; Miura, T; Yamamoto, S; Tsugane, S. Plasma isoflavone level and subsequent risk of breast cancer among Japanese women: a nested case-control study from the Japan Public Health Center-based prospective study group. *J. Clin. Oncol.,* 2008 26, 1677-1683.

[55] Lizardi-Cervera, J; Cuellar-Gamboa, L; Motola-Kuba, D. Focal nodular hyperplasia and hepatic adenoma: a review. *Ann. Hepatol.,* 2006 5, 206-211.

[56] Baum, JK; Bookstein, JJ; Holtz, F; Klein, EW. Possible association between benign hepatomas and oral contraceptives. *Lancet,* 1973 2, 926-929.

[57] Baek, S; Sloane, CE; Futterman, SC. Benign liver cell adenoma associated with use of oral contraceptive agents. *Ann. Surg.,* 1976 183, 239-242.

[58] Chen, YJ; Chen, PJ; Lee, MC; Yeh, SH; Hsu, MT; Lin, CH. Chromosomal analysis of hepatic adenoma and focal nodular hyperplasia by comparative genomic hybridization. *Genes Chromosomes Cancer,* 2002 35, 138-143.

[59] Shimizu, I; Yasuda, M; Mizobuchi, Y; Ma, YR; Liu, F; Shiba, M; Horie, T; Ito, S. Suppressive effect of oestradiol on chemical hepatocarcinogenesis in rats. *Gut,* 1998 42, 112-119.

[60] Yager, JD, Jr.; Yager, R. Oral contraceptive steroids as promoters of hepatocarcinogenesis in female Sprague-Dawley rats. *Cancer Res.,* 1980 40, 3680-3685.

[61] Cameron, R; Imaida, K; Ito, N. Promotive effects of ethinyl estradiol in hepatocarcinogenesis initiated by diethylnitrosamine in male rats. *Gann,* 1981 72, 339-340.

[62] Wanless, IR; Medline, A. Role of estrogens as promoters of hepatic neoplasia. *Lab. Invest,* 1982 46, 313-320.

[63] Heldring, N; Pike, A; Andersson, S; Matthews, J; Cheng, G; Hartman, J; Tujague, M; Strom, A; Treuter, E; Warner, M; Gustafsson, JA. Estrogen receptors: how do they signal and what are their targets. *Physiol. Rev.,* 2007 87, 905-931.

[64] Alvaro, D; Mancino, MG; Onori, P; Franchitto, A; Alpini, G; Francis, H; Glaser, S; Gaudio, E. Estrogens and the pathophysiology of the biliary tree. *World J. Gastroenterol.,* 2006 12, 3537-3545.

[65] Wang, AG; Lee, KY; Kim, SY; Choi, JY; Lee, KH; Kim, WH; Wang, HJ; Kim, JM; Park, MG; Yeom, YI; Kim, NS; Yu, DY; Lee, DS. The expression of estrogen receptors in hepatocellular carcinoma in Korean patients. *Yonsei Med. J.,* 2006 47, 811-816.

[66] Ohnishi, S; Murakami, T; Moriyama, T; Mitamura, K; Imawari, M. Androgen and estrogen receptors in hepatocellular carcinoma and in the surrounding noncancerous liver tissue. *Hepatology,* 1986 6, 440-443.

[67] Kohigashi, K; Fukuda, Y; Imura, H. Estrogen receptors in hepatocellular carcinoma: is endocrine therapy for hepatocellular carcinoma likely to be effective? *Gastroenterol. Jpn,* 1987 22, 322-330.

[68] Eagon, PK; Francavilla, A; DiLeo, A; Elm, MS; Gennari, L; Mazzaferro, V; Colella, G; Van Thiel, DH; Strazl, TE. Quantitation of estrogen and androgen receptors in hepatocellular carcinoma and adjacent normal human liver. *Dig. Dis. Sci.,* 1991 36, 1303-1308.

[69] Iavarone, M; Lampertico, P; Seletti, C; Francesca Donato, M; Ronchi, G; del Ninno, E; Colombo, M. The clinical and pathogenetic significance of estrogen receptor-beta expression in chronic liver diseases and liver carcinoma. *Cancer,* 2003 98, 529-534.

[70] Friedman, MA; Demanes, DJ; Hoffman, PG, Jr. Hepatomas: hormone receptors and therapy. *Am. J. Med.* 1982 73, 362-366.

[71] Iqbal, MJ; Wilkinson, ML; Johnson, PJ; Williams, R. Sex steroid receptor proteins in foetal, adult and malignant human liver tissue. *Br. J. Cancer,* 1983 48, 791-796.

[72] Liu, WH; Yeh, SH; Lu, CC; Yu, SL; Chen, HY; Lin, CY; Chen, DS; Chen, PJ. MicroRNA-18a prevents estrogen receptor-alpha expression, promoting proliferation of hepatocellular carcinoma cells. *Gastro-enterology,* 2009 136, 683-693.

[73] Villa, E; Camellini, L; Dugani, A; Zucchi, F; Grottola, A; Merighi, A; Buttafoco, P; Losi, L; Manenti, F. Variant estrogen receptor messenger RNA species detected in human primary hepatocellular carcinoma. *Cancer Res.,* 1995 55, 498-500.

[74] Castles, CG; Fuqua, SA; Klotz, DM; Hill, SM. Expression of a constitutively active estrogen receptor variant in the estrogen receptor-negative BT-20 human breast cancer cell line. *Cancer Res.,* 1993 53, 5934-5939.

[75] Villa, E; Colantoni, A; Camma, C; Grottola, A; Buttafoco, P; Gelmini, R; Ferretti, I; Manenti, F. Estrogen receptor classification for hepatocellular carcinoma: comparison with clinical staging systems. *J. Clin. Oncol.,* 2003 21, 441-446.

[76] Villa, E; Colantoni, A; Grottola, A; Ferretti, I; Buttafoco, P; Bertani, H; De Maria, N; Manenti, F. Variant estrogen receptors and their role in liver disease. *Mol. Cell Endocrinol.,* 2002 193, 65-69.

[77] Villa, E; Dugani, A; Moles, A; Camellini, L; Grottola, A; Buttafoco, P; Merighi, A; Ferretti, I; Esposito, P; Miglioli, L; Bagni, A; Troisi, R; De Hemptinne, B; Praet, M; Callea, F; Manenti, F. Variant liver estrogen receptor transcripts already occur at an early stage of chronic liver disease. *Hepatology,* 1998 27, 983-988.

[78] Villa, E; Dugani, A; Fantoni, E; Camellini, L; Buttafoco, P; Grottola, A; Pompei, G; De Santis, M; Ferrari, A; Manenti, F. Type of estrogen receptor determines response to antiestrogen therapy. *Cancer Res.,* 1996 56, 3883-3885.

[79] Villa, E; Moles, A; Ferretti, I; Buttafoco, P; Grottola, A; Del Buono, M; De Santis, M; Manenti, F. Natural history of inoperable hepatocellular carcinoma: estrogen receptors' status in the tumor is the strongest prognostic factor for survival. *Hepatology,* 2000 32, 233-238.

[80] Farinati, F; Cardin, R; Bortolami, M; Grottola, A; Manno, M; Colantoni, A; Villa, E. Estrogens receptors and oxidative damage in the liver. *Mol. Cell Endocrinol.,* 2002 193, 85-88.

[81] Han, J; Ding, L; Yuan, B; Yang, X; Wang, X; Li, J; Lu, Q; Huang, C; Ye, Q. Hepatitis B virus X protein and the estrogen receptor variant lacking exon 5 inhibit estrogen receptor signaling in hepatoma cells. *Nucleic. Acids. Res.,* 2006 34, 3095-3106.

[82] Mantovani, A; Allavena, P; Sica, A; Balkwill, F. Cancer-related inflammation. *Nature* 2008 454, 436-444.

[83] Karin, M; Lawrence, T; Nizet, V. Innate immunity gone awry: linking microbial infections to chronic inflammation and cancer. *Cell,* 2006 124, 823-835.

[84] Lin, WW; Karin, M. A cytokine-mediated link between innate immunity, inflammation, and cancer. *J. Clin. Invest.,* 2007 117, 1175-1183.

[85] Karin, M. Nuclear factor-kappaB in cancer development and progression. *Nature,* 2006 441, 431-436.

[86] Sun, B; Karin, M. NF-kappaB signaling, liver disease and hepato-protective agents. *Oncogene,* 2008 27, 6228-6244.

[87] Sakurai, T; He, G; Matsuzawa, A; Yu, GY; Maeda, S; Hardiman, G; Karin, M. Hepatocyte necrosis induced by oxidative stress and IL-1 alpha release mediate carcinogen-induced compensatory proliferation and liver tumorigenesis. *Cancer Cell,* 2008 14, 156-165.

[88] Pikarsky, E; Porat, RM; Stein, I; Abramovitch, R; Amit, S; Kasem, S; Gutkovich-Pyest, E; Urieli-Shoval, S; Galun, E; Ben-Neriah, Y. NF-kappaB functions as a tumour promoter in inflammation-associated cancer. *Nature,* 2004 431, 461-466.

[89] Maeda, S; Kamata, H; Luo, JL; Leffert, H; Karin, M. IKKbeta couples hepatocyte death to cytokine-driven compensatory proliferation that promotes chemical hepatocarcinogenesis. *Cell,* 2005 121, 977-990.

[90] Naugler, WE; Sakurai, T; Kim, S; Maeda, S; Kim, K; Elsharkawy, AM; Karin, M. Gender disparity in liver cancer due to sex differences in MyD88-dependent IL-6 production. *Science,* 2007 317, 121-124.

[91] Pfeilschifter, J; Koditz, R; Pfohl, M; Schatz, H. Changes in proinflammatory cytokine activity after menopause. *Endocr. Rev.*, 2002 23, 90-119.

[92] Rachon, D; Mysliwska, J; Suchecka-Rachon, K; Wieckiewicz, J; Mysliwski, A. Effects of oestrogen deprivation on interleukin-6 production by peripheral blood mononuclear cells of postmenopausal women. *J. Endocrinol.*, 2002 172, 387-395.

[93] Parsons, CJ; Takashima, M; Rippe, RA. Molecular mechanisms of hepatic fibrogenesis. *J Gastroenterol Hepatol*, 2007 22, S79-84.

[94] Poli, G. Pathogenesis of liver fibrosis: role of oxidative stress. *Mol. Aspects Med.*, 2000 21, 49-98.

[95] Lacort, M; Leal, AM; Liza, M; Martin, C; Martinez, R; Ruiz-Larrea, MB. Protective effect of estrogens and catecholestrogens against peroxidative membrane damage in vitro. *Lipids,* 1995 30, 141-146.

[96] Omoya, T; Shimizu, I; Zhou, Y; Okamura, Y; Inoue, H; Lu, G; Itonaga, M; Honda, H; Nomura, M; Ito, S. Effects of idoxifene and estradiol on NF-kappaB activation in cultured rat hepatocytes undergoing oxidative stress. *Liver,* 2001 21, 183-191.

[97] Inoue, H; Shimizu, I; Lu, G; Itonaga, M; Cui, X; Okamura, Y; Shono, M; Honda, H; Inoue, S; Muramatsu, M; Ito, S. Idoxifene and estradiol enhance antiapoptotic activity through estrogen receptor-beta in cultured rat hepatocytes. *Dig. Dis. Sci.,* 2003 48, 570-580.

[98] Yasuda, M; Shimizu, I; Shiba, M; Ito, S. Suppressive effects of estradiol on dimethylnitrosamine-induced fibrosis of the liver in rats. *Hepatology,* 1999 29, 719-727.

[99] Shimizu, I; Mizobuchi, Y; Yasuda, M; Shiba, M; Ma, YR; Horie, T; Liu, F; Ito, S. Inhibitory effect of oestradiol on activation of rat hepatic stellate cells in vivo and in vitro. *Gut,* 1999 44, 127-136.

[100] Lu, G; Shimizu, I; Cui, X; Itonaga, M; Tamaki, K; Fukuno, H; Inoue, H; Honda, H; Ito, S. Antioxidant and antiapoptotic activities of idoxifene and estradiol in hepatic fibrosis in rats. *Life Sci.,* 2004 74, 897-907.

[101] Poynard, T; Mathurin, P; Lai, CL; Guyader, D; Poupon, R; Tainturier, MH; Myers, RP; Muntenau, M; Ratziu, V; Manns, M; Vogel, A; Capron, F; Chedid, A; Bedossa, P. A comparison of fibrosis progression in chronic liver diseases. *J. Hepatol.,* 2003 38, 257-265.

[102] Zarski, JP; Marcellin, P; Leroy, V; Trepo, C; Samuel, D; Ganne-Carrie, N; Barange, K; Canva, V; Doffoel, M; Cales, P. Characteristics of patients with chronic hepatitis B in France: predominant frequency of HBe antigen negative cases. *J. Hepatol.,* 2006 45, 355-360.

[103] Iloeje, UH; Yang, HI; Su, J; Jen, CL; You, SL; Chen, CJ. Predicting cirrhosis risk based on the level of circulating hepatitis B viral load. *Gastroenterology,* 2006 130, 678-686.

[104] Lefkowitch, JH; Schiff, ER; Davis, GL; Perrillo, RP; Lindsay, K; Bodenheimer, HC Jr; Balart, LA; Ortego, TJ; Payne, J; Dienstag, JL; Gibas, A; Jacobson, IM; Tamburro, CH; Carey, W; Obrien, C; Sampliner, R; Vanthiel, DH; Feit, D; Albrecht, J; Meschievitz, C; Sanghvi, B; Vaughan, RD. Pathological diagnosis of chronic hepatitis C: a multicenter comparative study with chronic hepatitis B. The Hepatitis Interventional Therapy Group. *Gastroenterology,* 1993 104, 595-603.

[105] Czaja, AJ; Carpenter, HA. Sensitivity, specificity, and predictability of biopsy interpretations in chronic hepatitis. *Gastroenterology,* 1993 105, 1824-1832.

[106] Moriya, K; Fujie, H; Shintani, Y; Yotsuyanagi, H; Tsutsumi, T; Ishibashi, K; Matsuura, Y; Kimura, S; Miyamura, T; Koike, K. The core protein of hepatitis C virus induces hepatocellular carcinoma in transgenic mice. *Nat. Med.,* 1998 4, 1065-1067.

[107] Kim, CM; Koike, K; Saito, I; Miyamura, T; Jay, G. HBx gene of hepatitis B virus induces liver cancer in transgenic mice. *Nature* 1991 351, 317-320.

[108] Wu, BK; Li, CC; Chen, HJ; Chang, JL; Jeng, KS; Chou, CK; Hsu, MT; Tsai, TF. Blocking of G1/S transition and cell death in the regenerating liver of Hepatitis B virus X protein transgenic mice. *Biochem. Biophys. Res. Commun.,* 2006 340, 916-928.

[109] Oien, KA; Moffat, D; Curry, GW; Dickson, J; Habeshaw, T; Mills, PR; MacSween, RN. Cirrhosis with steatohepatitis after adjuvant tamoxifen. *Lancet,* 1999 353, 36-37.

[110] Van Hoof, M; Rahier, J; Horsmans, Y. Tamoxifen-induced steatohepatitis. *Ann. Intern. Med.,* 1996 124, 855-856.

[111] Nemoto, Y; Toda, K; Ono, M; Fujikawa-Adachi, K; Saibara, T; Onishi, S; Enzan, H; Okada, T; Shizuta, Y. Altered expression of fatty acid-metabolizing enzymes in aromatase-deficient mice. *J. Clin. Invest.,* 2000 105, 1819-1825.

[112] Weston, SR; Leyden, W; Murphy, R; Bass, NM; Bell, BP; Manos, MM; Terrault, NA. Racial and ethnic distribution of nonalcoholic fatty liver in persons with newly diagnosed chronic liver disease. *Hepatology,* 2005 41, 372-379.

[113] Jonas, S; Bechstein, WO; Heinze, T; Kling, N; Lobeck, H; Tullius, SG; Steinmueller, T; Neuhaus, P. Female sex hormone receptor status in advanced hepatocellular carcinoma and outcome after surgical resection. *Surgery,* 1997 121, 456-461.

[114] Nagasue, N; Kohno, H; Chang, YC; Yamanoi, A; Nakamura, T; Yukaya, H; Hayashi, T. Clinicopathologic comparisons between estrogen receptor-positive and -negative hepatocellular carcinomas. *Ann. Surg.,* 1990 212, 150-154.

[115] Shen, L; Ahuja, N; Shen, Y; Habib, NA; Toyota, M; Rashid, A; Issa, JP. DNA methylation and environmental exposures in human hepatocellular carcinoma. *J. Natl. Cancer Inst.,* 2002 94, 755-761.

[116] Pacchioni, D; Papotti, M; Andorno, E; Bonino, F; Mondardini, A; Oliveri, F; Brunetto, M; Bussolati, G; Negro, F. Expression of estrogen receptor mRNA in tumorous and non-tumorous liver tissue as detected by in situ hybridization. *J. Surg. Oncol. Suppl.,* 1993 3, 14-17.

[117] Krek, A; Grun, D; Poy, MN; Wolf, R; Rosenberg, L; Epstein, EJ; MacMenamin, P; da Piedade, I; Gunsalus, KC; Stoffel, M; Rajewsky, N. Combinatorial microRNA target predictions. *Nat. Genet,* 2005 37, 495-500.

[118] Lewis, BP; Burge, CB; Bartel, DP. Conserved seed pairing, often flanked by adenosines, indicates that thousands of human genes are microRNA targets. *Cell* 2005 120, 15-20.

[119] Almog, Y; Klein, A; Adler, R; Laub, O; Tur-Kaspa, R. Estrogen suppresses hepatitis B virus expression in male athymic mice transplanted with HBV transfected Hep G-2 cells. *Antiviral. Res.,* 1992 19, 285-293.

[120] Di Maio, M; Daniele, B; Pignata, S; Gallo, C; De Maio, E; Morabito, A; Piccirillo, MC; Perrone, F. Is human hepatocellular carcinoma a hormone-responsive tumor? *World J. Gastroenterol.,* 2008 14, 1682-1689.

[121] Tamoxifen for early breast cancer: an overview of the randomised trials. Early Breast Cancer Trialists' Collaborative Group. *Lancet,* 1998 351, 1451-1467.

[122] Simonetti, RG; Liberati, A; Angiolini, C; Pagliaro, L. Treatment of hepatocellular carcinoma: a systematic review of randomized controlled trials. *Ann. Oncol.,* 1997 8, 117-136.

[123] Mathurin, P; Rixe, O; Carbonell, N; Bernard, B; Cluzel, P; Bellin, MF; Khayat, D; Opolon, P; Poynard, T. Review article: Overview of medical treatments in unresectable hepatocellular carcinoma--an impossible meta-analysis? *Aliment. Pharmacol. Ther.,* 1998 12, 111-126.

[124] Llovet, JM; Bruix, J. Systematic review of randomized trials for unresectable hepatocellular carcinoma: Chemoembolization improves survival. *Hepatology,* 2003 37, 429-442.

[125] Nowak, AK; Stockler, MR; Chow, PK; Findlay, M. Use of tamoxifen in advanced-stage hepatocellular carcinoma. A systematic review. *Cancer,* 2005 103, 1408-1414.

[126] Tamoxifen in treatment of hepatocellular carcinoma: a randomised controlled trial. CLIP Group (Cancer of the Liver Italian Programme). *Lancet,* 1998 352, 17-20.

[127] Cameron, R; Imaida, K; Ito, N. Promotive effects of deoxycholic acid on hepatocarcinogenesis initiated by diethylnitrosamine in male rats. *Gann,* 1981 72, 635-636.

[128] Vickers, AE; Nelson, K; McCoy, Z; Lucier, GW. Changes in estrogen receptor, DNA ploidy, and estrogen metabolism in rat hepatocytes during a two-stage model for hepatocarcinogenesis using 17 alpha-ethinylestradiol as the promoting agent. *Cancer Res.,* 1989 49, 6512-6520.

[129] He, L; Thomson, JM; Hemann, MT; Hernando-Monge, E; Mu, D; Goodson, S; Powers, S; Cordon-Cardo, C; Lowe, SW; Hannon, GJ; Hammond, SM. A microRNA polycistron as a potential human oncogene. *Nature,* 2005 435, 828-833.

In: Estrogens
Editors: V. Thompson and A. Watson

ISBN 978-1-62081-747-6
© 2012 Nova Science Publishers, Inc.

Chapter 5

POST-TRANSCRIPTIONAL EFFECTS OF ESTROGENS ON GENE EXPRESSION: MESSENGER RNA STABILITY AND TRANSLATION REGULATED BY MICRORNAS AND OTHER FACTORS

Nancy H. Ing[*]
Texas A&M University,
Departments of Animal Science and Veterinary
Integrative Biosciences,
College Station, Texas, US

ABSTRACT

Estrogens exert powerful effects on physiology by regulating gene expression. Their effects on the transcriptional activities of genes are well described in the literature. However, estrogens are also the hormones that are best known for post-transcriptional gene regulation. With the combination of transcriptional and post-transcriptional regulation, gene expression can be rapidly and powerfully controlled to maximize the utility of genomic information throughout the long lives of vertebrate animals. For some cell responses, up to 50% of the genes with altered expression are the result of changes in the stabilities of the messenger

---

[*] Nancy H. Ing, D.V.M, Ph.D, Associate Professor. ning@cvm.tamu.edu

RNAs (mRNAs). For many genes including the estrogen receptor alpha (ER) gene, post-transcriptional regulation is the primary mode of alteration of expression. This indicates that post-transcriptional gene regulation is critical to estrogen actions because the ER protein determines the estrogen-responsiveness of animal tissues to a large extent. Estrogens have been shown to regulate the expression of certain genes by greatly altering the stabilities of mRNAs, including stabilizing ER mRNA. This effect may be ancient as it appears to be conserved from mammals to fish and frogs. Some studies have identified unique proteins that are induced by estrogens to bind and protect specific mRNAs from degradation. Recently, hundreds of microRNAs have been discovered and are estimated to actively regulate about one third of protein-encoding mRNAs. MicroRNAs associate with proteins in complexes on mRNAs, where they usually destabilize the mRNA or block its translation. Estrogens regulate the expression of microRNA genes in responsive tissues during normal physiology and disease processes. Other cell signals alter the expression of certain microRNAs that affect ER gene expression. Elucidation of the molecular mechanisms responsible for these post-transcriptional effects is certain to reveal novel molecular targets for therapeutic control of estrogen actions.

INTRODUCTION

Estrogens are a family of hormones that potently regulate reproductive, cardiovascular, bone, brain and other physiology in vertebrates by altering gene expression [Tsai et al., 1998]. Estrogens regulate gene expression on several levels. The mechanisms by which estrogen regulates the rate of transcription of genes (messenger RNA (mRNA) synthesis) are well described. However, concentrations of mRNAs are also dependent upon their rates of degradation. Posttranscriptional regulation of gene expression at the level of mRNA stability is rapidly being recognized as a powerful and widespread phenomenon [Tsai et al., 1998; Watson et al., 2007]. For some cell responses, up to 50% of the changes in concentrations of mRNAs are the result of changes in the stabilities of the mRNAs [Cheadle et al., 2005]. There are also effects on the rates of translation of mRNAs with little or no change in mRNA concentration. For the sake of space, this chapter does not address post-translational effects of estrogens on gene expression. Estrogens are the hormones best known for post-transcriptional regulation of gene expression. For many genes, including that of estrogen receptor alpha (ER), post-transcriptional regulation is the primary mode of regulation of gene expression

[Ing, 2005a]. In the following review, we will use the post-transcriptional regulation of the expression of the ER gene as an example because (1) the ER protein transduces the majority of estrogen effects, (2) the ER gene is predominantly regulated post-transcriptionally, and (3) several different post-transcriptional mechanisms regulate the expression of the ER gene. The post-transcriptional regulation of the ER gene is likely to be common to a set of mRNAs (an "mRNA regulon") that are coordinately expressed but remain to be identified [Keene, 2007].

Post-transcriptional regulation of mRNA stabilities is similar to transcriptional regulation of genes, but with cytoplasmic trans-acting factors (including proteins and microRNAs) acting on cis-elements within the mRNAs. Most of the information controlling translation efficiency and mRNA stability is carried within the 5' and 3' untranslated regions (UTRs) of the mRNA, respectively. Typically, 5'UTRs are short (100 to 200 bases long) and are involved with ribosome loading and the initiation of translation. In contrast, the 3' UTRs of mRNAs can be quite extensive (500 to > 5,000 bases) and in many cases the 3' UTR sequences compose the majority of the mRNA. For example, the 6351 base long ER mRNA of the sheep carries 4354 bases of 3'UTR [Mitchell and Ing, 2003]. 3'UTRs regulate mRNA stability and are usually encoded in only one exon so they are not subject to alternative splicing [Nagy and Maquat, 1998]. Although mRNAs are often graphically represented as straight lines, mRNAs adopt complex secondary and tertiary structures by the intramolecular pairing of bases. The 3'UTRs of mRNAs are unique in that they are not subjected to passage of ribosomes, so their secondary and tertiary structures are likely to be more stable than those in other mRNA regions. While overall conservation of 3' UTR sequences of mRNA homologs between species is lower than in coding sequences, there are relatively large (> 500 base long) regions within 3' UTRs that are highly conserved across species [Mitchell and Ing, 2003]. This conservation of sequences in non-coding RNA regions implies that the sequences have important function(s) and the primary function of 3' UTR sequences is the regulation of mRNA stability.

The transacting factors (protein and microRNAs) that bind mRNA cis-elements determine the function and fate of the mRNA. ER mRNA is similar to a lot of other mRNAs encoding hormone receptors in that it is inherently unstable because its very long 3'UTR that carries destabilizing mRNA cis-elements such as the A+U Rich Element (ARE) [Chen and Shyu, 1995; Mitchell and Ing, 2003]. Sheep and human ER mRNAs carry 10 and 14 putative AREs, respectively, and all are in the 3'UTR [Kenealy et al., 2000; Mitchell and Ing, 2003]. Transfer of the 3' UTRs of ER mRNA to other mRNAs destabilizes those mRNAs. AREs destabilize mRNAs by binding destabilizing factors such as A + U-rich binding factor 1 p37 (AUF1p37) and tristetraprolin which direct the mRNA to exosomes, where mRNAs are degraded [Zhao et al., 2000; Parker and Song, 2004; Mukherjee et al., 2002]. There are also examples of mRNA stabilizing proteins such as HuR which, in response to cell signals, competitively bind AREs and prevent destabilization [Sengupta et al., 2003; Lasa et al., 2000; Wilson et al., 2001; Chen et al., 2002]. In every cell, the lifespan of an mRNA depends upon the balance of these influences. The discovery of microRNAs as a major class of post-transcriptional regulators of gene expression in animal tissues has revolutionized the field of gene expression. Whether microRNAs interact with destabilizing proteins like AUF1p37 in the same or different ribonucleoprotein complexes remains to be determined. Estrogens regulate mRNA stabilities, mRNA binding proteins, and microRNAs, as discussed below. Knowledge gained in this rapidly emerging field of post-transcriptional gene regulation will greatly improve our understanding of estrogen actions in normal and pathological tissues.

Estrogen influence and ER regulation are important in numerous aspects of normal physiology as well as in the development of hormone-dependent diseases. For example, the incidences of breast and uterine cancers and endometriosis in women are related to their exposure to estrogens [McKean-Cowdin et al., 2001; Gurates and Bulun, 2003]. The incidence of breast cancer (carcinoma) has doubled worldwide over the last 20 years and it will occur in 1 out of 9 women in the USA [Yan et al., 2008]. The ability of breast tumors to respond to estrogens is dependent upon the expression of ER. Breast cancer cases with the worst prognosis and advanced disease typically lack ER protein and do not respond to treatment with Selective Estrogen Receptor Modulators (SERMs) drugs like tamoxifen and raloxifene [Jordan and O'Malley, 2007]. Uterine leiomyomas (also called uterine fibroids) are non-malignant myometrial cancers that are remarkably common in women of reproductive ages, with autopsy studies indicating their presence in more than 75% of those women [Cramer and Patel, 1990]. In about 25% of women of reproductive ages, leiomyomas cause pain, bleeding and infertility. Leiomyomas are the most common reason for hysterectomies. Leiomyomas have increased concentrations of estrogen-responsive genes, including the ER gene, compared to neighboring normal myometrium. Recent studies have identified alterations in expression microRNA genes that correlate with these estrogen-dependent diseases and might be useful for prognoses [Wang et al., 2007b; Yan et al., 2008]. Studies are beginning to unravel the post-transcriptional processes by which estrogens act, which probably reflect alterations in the compositions of ribonucleoprotein complexes on mRNAs. Elucidation of the molecular mechanisms responsible for estrogen-dependent physiology and disease processes is likely to provide novel targets and approaches for therapies.

ESTROGENS STABILIZE AND DESTABILIZE SPECIFIC mRNAS

Expression of the ER gene in the uterus is tightly regulated by steroid hormones from the ovary. In the luteal phases of estrous and menstrual cycles, progesterone down-regulates ER gene expression [Miller et al., 1979]. The subsequent preovulatory surge of estrogen up-regulates concentrations of ER mRNA and protein to restore estrogen responsiveness to the uterus, which is critical to its support of developing embryos [Ing, 1999; Moore et al., 1983]. Estrogen up-regulation of ER gene expression occurs in several tissues of vertebrate species ranging from fish to mammals [Ing, 1999; Friend et al., 1997; Rodriguez-Pinon et al., 2005]. In our animal model, the ovariectomized ewe, one physiological dose of estradiol up-regulates ER mRNA abundance in the uterus by 5-fold in 24 h [Ing and Ott, 1999; Mitchell and Ing, 2003]. ER was required for the up-regulation because SERM drugs blocked the effect [Robertson et al., 2001; Farnell and Ing, 2003c; Farnell and Ing, 2003b; Farnell and Ing, 2003a]. Nuclear runoff experiments detected no increase in the rate of transcription of the ER gene. However, both pulse-chase and transcription inhibitor experiments demonstrated that estradiol treatment enhanced ER mRNA stability.

The mechanism of estrogen stabilization of ER mRNA was investigated to identify the cis-elements (mRNA sequences) and transacting factors (binding proteins) involved. Using a cell-free assay for mRNA stability, the ER mRNA sequences responsible for estradiol-enhanced stability were localized within the 3' UTR. The mRNA stability assay employed cytosolic extracts from uteri of control and estradiol-treated ewes. The assay reproduced the mRNA specificity and magnitude of the stabilization of ER mRNA in the uterus of the ewe. Extensive studies identified two 82 base long Minimal Estrogen Modulated Stability Sequences (MEMSS) within the 4354 base long 3'UTR of ER mRNA [Mitchell and Ing, 2003]. Both MEMSS contained a 10 base long U-rich element (URE) that was predicted to be positioned on the ends of stem-loop structures [Mitchell and Ing, 2003]. Also, both MEMSS conferred E2-

enhanced stability when transferred to heterologous RNAs. The stabilizing factor(s) that bind MEMSS appears to be proteinaceous because proteinase K or 70°C heat treatment eliminated the enhanced stability of ER mRNA in uterine extracts from estradiol-treated ewes [Mitchell and Ing, 2003]. UV-crosslinking was used to detect four MEMSS-binding proteins that were induced by estradiol treatment. The predominant, estradiol-induced binding protein immunoprecipitated with antiserum to AUF1. The size of the binding protein identified it as AUF1p45. AUF1 mRNA is alternatively spliced to translate four protein isoforms: AUF1p37, -p40, -p42, and -p45 [Wagner et al., 1998]. All bind AREs, but AUF1p40 and -p45 carry an mRNA stabilizing domain while the AUF1p37 and -p42 isoforms are associated with destabilized mRNAs [Sela-Brown et al., 2000; Loflin et al., 1999; Xu et al., 2001]. In vivo estradiol treatment increased AUF1p45 concentrations (probably non-phosphorylated) 6-fold in the uterine extracts [Ing et al., 2008]. Recombinant AUF1p45 stabilized ER mRNA in the mRNA stability assay with uterine extracts. A model for the mechanism of ER mRNA stabilization by estrogens is presented in Figure 1.

In it, an estrogen up-regulates AUF1p45 which, along with other proteins and perhaps microRNAs, binds the two MEMSS within the 3'UTR of ER mRNA to form ribonucleoprotein complexes that stabilize ER mRNA.While this mechanism was discovered in sheep uteri, it is likely to operate in other species and tissues to up-regulate ER mRNA and protein concentrations. The mechanistic work with the sheep uterus complements studies of other mRNAs.

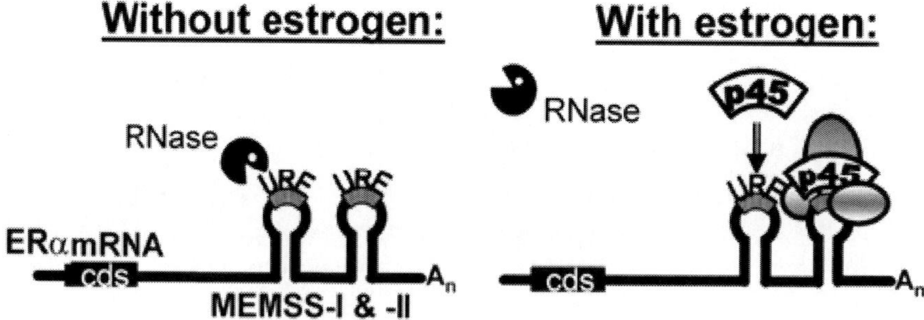

Figure 1. Model for E2 induction of a stabilizing ribonucleoprotein complex (RNP) on ER mRNA. The cartoon mRNA shows the coding of ER sequence (cds) 5' to the extensive 3'UTR. Within the 3'UTR, two 82 base Minimal Estradiol (E2) Modulated Stability Sequences (MEMSS) carry 10 base U-rich sequences (UREs) on stem loop structures. Estrogen induces binding of proteins to form a stabilizing RNP composed of proteins (AUF1p45 and shaded mRNA to protect it from ribonuclease (RNase).circles) on ER.

In rat uteri, estradiol treatment increased AUF1p40 expression by stabilizing the mRNA encoding it [Arao et al., 2002]. Estradiol treatment also up-regulated expression of two immediate early genes, encoding Immediate Early Response 2 (IER2) and TNFAIP3 Interacting protein 2 (TNIP2). These were initially identified by screening for mRNAs bound by AUF1 proteins [Arao et al., 2004]. This data implies that estradiol treatment stabilizes a set of mRNAs in rat uteri. This is a common theme in post-transcriptional gene regulation and some call these sets of coordinately regulated mRNAs "RNA regulons" [Keene, 2007]. It is expected that future experiments will identify groups of estrogen-stabilized mRNAs. Most of the initial studies of estrogen effects on stabilities of mRNAs were performed in egg-laying animals [Dodson and Shapiro, 2002]. In the livers of male frogs treated with estradiol, the mRNA encoding vitellogenin is stabilized from having a half-life of 16 h to having one of 600 h. This is believed to occur in female frogs and other egg-laying species at the beginning of oogenesis. The mechanism is similar to the stabilization of ER mRNA in that estrogen induces a protein to bind vitellogenin mRNA on several sites within the 3' UTR. In the frog liver, estrogen induces production of the vigilin protein, which carries 15 RNA-binding domains [Cunningham et al., 2000]. The binding of vigilin to vitellogenin mRNA sterically blocks A(C/U)UGA sites that are susceptible to cleavage by an endonuclease named polysomal ribonuclease 1. Intriguingly, this endonuclease is also responsible for the concurrent destabilization of albumin mRNA in the livers of frogs treated with estradiol [Cunningham et al., 2001]. These estrogen-regulated posttranscriptional effects shift the gene expression program of the liver away from the production of serum proteins (such as albumin) and toward increased synthesis of proteins that will be packaged into eggs (such as vitellogenin).

There are numerous recent reports of estrogen-regulated stabilities of mRNAs in mammalian cells and tissues [Ing, 2005b]. One example with mechanistic information is the stabilization of luteinizing hormone receptor (LHR) in the granulosa cells within human and rat ovaries. Follicle stimulating hormone (FSH) followed by the preovulatory surge of estrogen increases LHR protein concentrations by stabilizing LHR mRNA [Wang et al., 2007a; Nair et al., 2008; Ikeda et al., 2008]. The stability of the LHR mRNA is inversely proportional to binding of a protein to sequence elements in the 3' UTR. The LHR mRNA binding protein was identified as mevalonate kinase, which was initially characterized for its role in cholesterol metabolism. The combination of FSH and estrogen influences down-regulate mevalonate kinase which, otherwise, would destabilize LHR mRNA. This action of mevalonate kinase in post-transcriptional regulation of LHR mRNA joins other examples of previously characterized metabolic enzymes that bind RNA and participate in post-transcriptional gene regulation [Kyrpides and Ouzounis, 1995; Ciesla, 2006]. These studies indicate the complexity of the interrelationships of gene products that participate in the regulation of vertebrate genes.

There are more and more intriguing examples of estrogens regulating of stabilities of mRNAs encoding critical gene products that await mechanistic information [Ing, 2005b]. The majority of examples of estrogen regulating mRNA stability involve stabilization in response to estrogen. In many cases, the regulation is tissue-specific. For example, in the mammalian pituitary, estrogen stabilizes some mRNAs, such as that encoding thyroid hormone releasing hormone receptor [el Meskini et al., 1997]. Other mRNAs, including that encoding the peptidylglycine alpha-amidating monooxygenase, are destabilized in the pituitary after estradiol treatment [Kimura et al., 1994]. Interestingly, one group reported that estradiol treatment destabilized ER mRNA in the MCF7 breast cancer cell line [Saceda et al., 1998]. The mechanism for destabilization of ER mRNA was not determined but could involve microRNAs, as discussed below. Comparisons of the molecular mechanisms by which estrogens regulate the stabilities of different mRNAs in various tissues may identify common or unique cis-elements and transacting factors. These could provide a way to predict and control the post-transcriptional effects of estrogen on gene regulation.

ESTROGENS AFFECT MRNA TRANSLATION

In many model systems, estrogens increase the rate of initiation of translation as well as the elongation rate of the nascent peptides. However, in most instances the effects are general and are not specific to one mRNA or a subset of mRNAs [Palmiter, 1972; Whelly and Barker, 1974]. There are a few exceptions that were published more than 20 years ago. In one example, estradiol treatment stimulated the synthesis of the ovalbumin protein in the chick oviduct while concentrations of ovalbumin mRNA decreased [Seaver, 1981]. This indicates that estradiol increased the rate of translation of ovalbumin mRNA and the effect appeared unique to that particular mRNA. The molecular mechanisms for the reported translational effects of estrogen are unknown.

However, recent evidence demonstrates that estrogen effects on the expression of microRNA genes and microRNAs can alter the translation of individual mRNAs in positive as well as negative manners, as discussed below.

ESTROGEN ACTIONS AND MICRORNAS

MicroRNAs – Biogenesis and Regulation of Gene Expression

MicroRNAs are an abundant class of non-coding RNAs. There are hundreds of microRNAs (~600 confirmed in humans) which range from 21 to 23 bases in length [Maziere and Enright, 2007]. MicroRNA sequences are very highly conserved across species. There are families of microRNAs that have related sequences and, in some cases, their genes are clustered on chromosomes and share coordinate expression in animal tissues. Primary transcripts of microRNAs are synthesized by RNA polymerase II or III [Lodish et al., 2008]. Microprocessor complexes containing the RNAse III-type endonuclease Drosha cleave the primary microRNA transcript to an approximately 60 base long RNA with hairpin structure called a pre-microRNA, which is exported to the cytoplasm. Pre-microRNAs are then cleaved by another RNAse III endonuclease, Dicer, which produces a double-stranded approximately 22 base long product. One strand is the mature microRNA, which is incorporated into the RNA-induced silencing complex (RISC) so that the microRNA can direct the actions of this effector complex to specific mRNAs by hybridizing to them [Jackson and Standart, 2007]. Each microRNA is predicted to bind and regulate an average of about 200 mRNAs. In this way, microRNAs are proposed to regulate 30 to 90% of mammalian mRNAs [Ioshikhes et al., 2007; Lodish et al., 2008].

MicroRNAs bind sequences within the 3' UTRs of mRNAs to regulate mRNA stability or translation. The complementary binding of a microRNA to a target mRNA is usually not complete. The 5' ends of microRNAs generally bind most strongly to the mRNA, with a 6- to 8- base long "seed" sequence beginning at the second base of the microRNA. There are often mismatches in the next 9 to 12 bases of the microRNA, followed by more base-pairing between bases 13 to 16 of the microRNA and the mRNA [Grimson et al., 2007]. Algorithms (MiRanda, TargetScan and PicTar) have been developed to predict microRNAs binding sites on mRNAs [Ioshikhes et al., 2007; Maziere and Enright, 2007].

The PicTar algorithm also takes into account sequence conservation of the predicted site on the target mRNA across species as further indication of function of the putative microRNA binding sites [Ioshikhes et al., 2007]. However, some microRNA sites in nonconserved regions have been shown to very effectively bind microRNAs that regulate the function of that mRNA [Baek et al., 2008]. There is growing evidence for cooperativity between microRNAs (similar or different) bound to neighboring sites, resulting in enhanced effects on the function of the mRNA [Grimson et al., 2007]. The effectiveness of microRNAs is also enhanced by flanking AU-rich regions [Grimson et al., 2007]. With increased understanding of microRNA interactions with mRNAs, we will be better able to predict and potentially utilize microRNA effects on gene expression.

The molecular mechanisms by which microRNAs regulate mRNA stability or the rate of mRNA translation are being actively studied. After the microRNA binds to the mRNA, it generally has one of two actions: destabilization of the mRNA or inhibition of translation [Jackson and Standart, 2007; Wu and Belasco, 2008]. In cases of mRNA destabilization, the microRNA decreases the concentrations of both the mRNA targeted as well as of the protein encoded by the mRNA. MicroRNAs that destabilize mRNA targets were originally thought to direct endonucleolytic cleavage by the RISC, as do short interfering RNAs [Jackson and Standart, 2007]. However, new evidence indicates that microRNAs can also induce rapid deadenylation of target mRNAs in animal cells, which then results in mRNA degradation [Wu and Belasco, 2008]. A recent study in animal cells indicated that the microRNAs that most powerfully down-regulate proteins also down-regulate the mRNAs encoding the proteins [Baek et al., 2008]. In the case of microRNAs inhibiting translation, the concentration of mRNA target remains unchanged while the concentration of the encoded protein decreases. MicroRNAs inhibit translation initiation by inhibiting recognition of the 5' cap of mRNA by ribosomes [Mathonnet et al., 2007]. The mode of microRNA binding to the mRNA may dictate whether the mRNA is destabilized or translation is repressed: more complete complementarity in binding may result in mRNA destabilization while less complementarity may lead to inhibition of translation [Saxena et al., 2003; Grimson et al., 2007; Maziere and Enright, 2007]. The actions of microRNAs are also dependent upon the proteins they associate with in ribonucleoprotein complexes [Jing et al., 2005; Bhattacharyya et al., 2006]. In addition, the binding of some proteins to mRNAs on sites near microRNA binding sites can prevent mRNA repression by the microRNA [Ketting, 2007; Kedde et al., 2007].

There is also a small but growing number of reports of microRNAs up-regulating gene expression, either by stabilizing mRNAs or by increasing mRNA translation rates [Krutzfeldt et al., 2005; Jackson and Standart, 2007]. The latter effect is apparent in quiescent cells and occurs by microRNAs recruiting Argonaut and other proteins to the mRNA [Jackson and Standart, 2007]. More experiments are required to discover the breadth of microRNA actions on gene expression in animal tissues.

Estrogens Regulate Expression of MicroRNA Genes in Responsive Tissues during Normal Physiology and Disease

Because of the importance of microRNAs in the regulation of gene expression, microRNA expression profiles are being studied in normal and pathological tissues [Landgraf et al., 2007; Liang et al., 2007; Hammond, 2006; Jiang et al., 2009]. For example, microRNA expression in human cancers is being evaluated to discern patterns for diagnostic and prognostic purposes [Jay et al., 2007; Lu et al., 2005; Lui et al., 2007; Boren et al., 2008]. Not surprisingly, since estrogens affect the expression of numerous protein-encoding genes, estrogens also affect the expression of numerous microRNA genes (Table 1).

All of the studies listed in Table 1 initially used microarray analyses and then confirmed altered concentrations of the microRNAs with real time PCR and/or Northern blotting. This increases the validity of the experimental results reported in Table 1. However, it also means that the data summarized in Table 1 are only a subset of the microRNAs that are regulated by estrogen and that the data are biased by the investigators' selection of the microRNAs chosen for confirmation by the second technique.

The data shown in Table 1 are compiled from studies in which animals or cells were treated directly with estradiol as well as from studies of animals and tissues that are known to have lesser or greater estrogen influence, as discussed below.

Estrogens regulate microRNA gene expression in tissue- and time-dependent manners. Regulation of microRNAs by estradiol treatment was directly tested in a fairly comprehensive study of zebrafish [Cohen et al., 2008]. Table 1 shows the four microRNAs up-regulated and four others down-regulated when whole fish were measured 24 h after treatment. The study went on to examine the microRNAs in specific tissues of the fish over a time course. Time dependent differences were found, such as down-regulation of dre-miR-26b concentrations by 40% at 12 h but return to baseline levels by 24 h after estradiol treatment. It is noteworthy that the ER protein concentrations peaked in the fish at 12 h post-treatment.

Table 1. Estrogen regulation of microRNAs in normal and pathological tissues. Selected data from studies using microarrays followed by confirmation with real time PCR and/or Northern blotting

miRNA	Estrogen regulation	Estrogen treatment or influence and tissue or cultured cells	Reference
Let7h	Up	Estradiol-treated zebrafish (whole body)	Cohen et al., 2008
122	Up		
196b	Up		
29b*	Up		
101a	Down		
130c	Down		
19a	Down		
460-5p	Down		
101a	Down	Estrogen-dominated uterus (mouse)	Chakrabarty et al., 2007
199a-3p	Down		
26a	Up	Estradiol-treated primary cultures of endometrial stromal cells (human)	Pan et al., 2007
20a	Down		
21	Down		
323	Up	Leiomyoma compared to myometrium (human)	Marsh et al., 2008
34a	Up		
139	Down		
Let7b	Up	Leiomyoma compared to myometrium (human)	Wang, et al., 2007
145	Up		
199a-3p	Up		
21	Up		
23b	Up		
26a	Up		
99a	Down		
29b	Down		
203	Down		
220	Down		
106a	Up	Estradiol-treated rats - mammary tissue undergoing carcinogenesis	Kovalchuk et al, 2007
129-3p	Up		
17-5p	Up		
20a	Up		
21	Up		
92	Up		
127	Down		
21	Up	Breast tumors compared to normal mammary tissues (human)	Iorio et al., 2005
125b	Down		
145	Down		
21	Up	Breast tumors compared to normal mammary tissues (human)	Yan et al., 2008
497	Down		
206	Down	Estradiol-treated MCF7 breast cancer cell line (human)	Adams et al., 2007

It is also important to note that microRNAs are very highly conserved. For example, the zebrafish dre-miR-26b mentioned is identical to the human hsa-miR-26a except for two bases on the 3'end. In primary cultures of human endometrial stromal cells, estradiol treatment regulated the expression of three microRNA genes while concurrent treatment with the SERM ICI 182,780 blocked the effect [Pan et al., 2007]. In rats treated long-term with estradiol, expression of six microRNA genes was up-regulated and one other was down-regulated in the mammary tissue that was undergoing carcinogenesis [Kovalchuk et al., 2007]. For some of the other studies with results in Table 1, estrogen regulation of microRNAs was implied. For example, in the mouse uterus, tissues were compared between animals in estrogen-dominated vs. progesterone-dominated phases of the estrous cycle [Chakrabarty et al., 2007]. Since miR-101a and -199a-3p concentrations were greater in the latter, we infer that estrogens may down-regulate them. This study identified cyclooxygenase 2 (COX2) mRNA as a target of miR-101a and -199a-3p and that these microRNAs inhibited COX2 mRNA translation in the mouse uterus during early pregnancy [Chakrabarty et al., 2007]. Microarray data also indicated that expression of miR-31 and -368 genes was lower in myometrial tissue from women during the estrogen-dominated follicular phase of the menstrual cycle, implying down-regulation by estrogens [Wang et al., 2007b]. Together, these data are an indication of the long-reaching effects of estrogens on microRNA gene expression in normal vertebrate animal tissues.

Estrogens also regulate microRNA gene expression in estrogen-dependent diseases. The latter include endometriosis, endometrial cancer, leiomyoma (uterine fibroids) and breast cancer. Microarray data indicated that expression of miR-20a, -21, and -26a genes, previously mentioned as being estradiol-regulated in endometrial stromal cells, was also deregulated in endometriotic tissue compared to normal endometrium [Pan et al., 2007]. In matched samples of endometrial cancer and normal endometrium from women, micro-array data indicated that miR-103, -107 and -185 concentrations were up-regulated while that of miR-let-7i was down-regulated [Boren et al., 2008]. In the case of leiomyomas, these tumors of the myometrium are well-known to have higher levels of estrogens as well as expression of estrogen-responsive genes compared to neighboring normal myometrium [Nowak, 2001]. Table 1 shows results from comparisions of matched leiomyoma and neighboring normal myometrial samples that detected several differentially expressed microRNAs [Wang et al., 2007b; Marsh et al., 2008]. Breast tumors are routinely characterized for treatment and prognosis by ER and proges-terone receptor (PR) protein immunohistochemistry [Mattie et al., 2006].

Tumors containing significant immunoreactivity for ER and PR proteins (ER+/PR+) are considered to be more differentiated (normal) and responsive to treatment with SERMs. It is important to note that as estrogens up-regulate gene expression, they also down-regulate concentrations of ER protein in the responsive tissues/cells as part of their transcriptional activation [Chu et al., 2007]. Because estrogens up-regulate PR gene expression, PR+ status is probably the best indicator that estrogen influence is dominant in a breast tumor sample. Results from three studies that compared microRNAs in breast tumors and related the data to the ER and PR protein status of the tumors are summarized in Table 1 [Iorio et al., 2005; Mattie et al., 2006; Foekens et al., 2008]. Microarray data from the first two studies agreed that microRNAs let-7c, 26a, 30a-5p, 30b and 30c were up-regulated in PR+ tumors compared to PR- tumors. The third study identified miR-22 and-34b as up-regulated in PR+ breast tumors compared to others [Foekens et al., 2008]. Intriguingly, all three studies identified only increases in microRNA concentrations (those named and others) in PR+ compared to PR- breast tumors, while no microRNA concentrations appeared to decrease. Differences in results between similar microRNA studies may be the result of individual differences in the women, the method or microarray platform used, or sampling technique (times of sampling, stage of the menstrual cycle, etc.). What is clear is that we need more good studies of microRNAs in human tissues, both during normal physiology and during the pathogenesis of estrogen-dependent diseases.

It is interesting that several microRNAs in Table 1 appear to be estrogen-regulated in more than one normal and/or pathological tissues. For example, miR-101 was down-regulated by estradiol treatment of zebrafish as well as during the estrogen-dominated phase of the estrous cycle in the uteri of mice [Chakrabarty et al., 2007; Cohen et al., 2008]. In addition, miR-26a concentrations were up-regulated by estradiol treatment in endometrial stromal cells in culture and were greater in leiomyoma compared to myometrium and in ER+/PR+ breast tumors compared to other tumors [Iorio et al., 2005; Pan et al., 2007; Wang et al., 2007b]. Concentrations of miR-21 appeared to be regulated by estrogens in five of the studies in Table 1. Concentrations of miR-21 were greater in leiomyomas and breast tumors compared to normal tissues as well as in mammary tissues of estradiol-treated rats [Yan et al., 2008; Kovalchuk et al., 2007; Wang et al., 2007b; Iorio et al., 2005]. It is noteworthy that high levels of miR-21 correlate to poor prognosis for breast cancer patients [Yan et al., 2008]. However, not all studies indicate the same direction of the microRNA gene's regulation by estrogen, either up or down. For example, estradiol treatment decreased concentrations of miR-21 in cultured endometrial stromal cells [Pan et al., 2007;]. Also, concentrations of miR-199a-3p were down-regulated in mouse uterus during the estrogen-dominated phase of the estrous cycle but were up-regulated in leiomyoma compared to normal myometrium. In conclusion, there are some consistent patterns for estrogen regulation of microRNA gene expression in vertebrate tissues. However, there are also some divergences that remain to be explained. Future research is needed to expand our understanding of how estrogens regulate the expression of microRNA genes in health and disease.

MicroRNAs Regulate ER Gene Expression and Estrogen Actions

While estrogens regulate the expression of microRNA genes, microRNAs also regulate the gene products that transduce the actions of estrogen in tissues: ER, cofactors, and kinase signaling cascades. Several studies demonstrated that microRNAs regulate expression of the ER gene. One study began with interest in microRNAs that had increased concentrations in ER-breast tumors compared to ER+ breast tumors [Iorio et al., 2005]. Among those microRNAs, the investigators focused on the few microRNAs that also had predicted binding sites within the 3'UTR of ER mRNA [Adams et al., 2007]. This lead to the discovery that experimentally altering the concentrations of miR-206 caused opposite effects on ER gene expression in MCF7 cells. The mechanism was by miR-206 destabilizing ER mRNA. Further studies demonstrated that estradiol treatment decreases concentrations of miR-206, leading to increased ER mRNA stability and ER protein concentrations. This describes a second mechanism by which estrogens post-transcriptionally up-regulate ER gene expression in addition to that described in the sheep uterus (Figure 1). Another group searching for microRNAs that regulate ER gene expression identified 12 microRNAs that were more highly expressed in ER- breast cancer cell lines compared to ER+ lines [Zhao et al., 2008]. These investigators predicted that miR-221 and -222 would target the 3'UTR of ER mRNA. By altering levels of the microRNAs in the MCF7 and T47D breast cancer cell lines, they demonstrated that miR-221 and -222 decreased ER protein but not mRNA concentrations, indicating that these two microRNAs inhibit translation of ER mRNA. Studies of a human pancreatic cancer cell line lead to the discovery that treatment with curcumin (a naturally occurring flavonoid that inhibits cancer growth) increased miR-22 and decreased miR-199a-3p concentrations [Sun et al., 2008]. Experimental up-regulation of miR-22 suppressed ER protein concentrations along with those of Sp1, which is a transcription factor that works with ER to activate transcription on many gene promoters that lack conventional estrogen-responsive elements. Thus, miR-22 appears to inhibit ER and ER/Sp1 responsive gene promoters by reducing the concentrations of those transcription factors. These examples show that several different microRNAs regulate the expression of the ER gene in a variety of tumor cells.

MicroRNAs can inhibit estrogen actions in ways other than decreasing ER protein concentrations. Phosphorylation of the ER protein is required for its function [Arnold et al., 1997; Vasudevan and Pfaff, 2008]. Phosphorylation is important for both the genomic actions of estrogens and the rapid, non-genomic effects of estrogens that involve kinase cascades [Watson et al., 2007]. We are just beginning to understand how microRNAs regulate phosphory-lation pathways in cells. In fibroblast cell lines, miR-199a-3p down-regulates extracellular signal-regulated kinase 2 (ERK2) [Kim et al., 2008]. Although estradiol treatment was not a part of that study, concen-rations of miR-199a-3p appeared to be down-regulated by estrogen in mouse uteri and were greater in leiomyomas compared to normal myometrium in women (Table 1). In another example, the expression of the miR-17-5p gene was inversely correlated to the expression of the Amplified In Breast cancer 1 (AIB1) gene in breast cancer cell lines [Hossain et al., 2006]. AIB1 is a coactivator that works with ER to activate transcription of responsive genes. AIB1 gene expression is up-regulated in many tumors including breast cancers. MiR-17-5p decreased the expression of the AIB1 gene by inhibiting AIB1 mRNA translation. Thus, miR-17-5p acts as a tumor suppressor by down-regulating AIB1 concentrations and estrogen signaling. Interestingly, miR-17-5p decreases both estrogen/ER-dependent and estrogen/ER-independent proliferation in the MCF7 breast cancer cell line [Hossain et al., 2006]. Increased knowledge about microRNA actions may lead to new therapies that utilize microRNAs to fight diseases such as cancer.

FUTURE THERAPEUTIC APPROACHES TO REGULATING POST-TRANSCRIPTIONAL ESTROGEN ACTIONS

Over the last decades, several therapies have been developed to control estrogen effects in humans in order to treat or prevent estrogen-dependent diseases. Because of that, there are several currently available drugs to modulate estrogen effects in vivo. From more general to specific,

Gonadotrophin Releasing Hormone (GnRH) agonists block gonadal steroid production and thereby estrogen and progesterone effects. More recently, aromatase inhibitors were developed to block estrogen production in all tissues of the body. Both GnRH agonists and aromatase inhibitors reduce all estrogen effects in the body, including the desirable ones that preserve bone, brain and circulatory system health. The SERMs modulate ER actions in a more tissue-specific manner. For example, treatment with the SERM raloxifene interferes with ER+ breast cancer growth while providing healthful estrogenic effects in bone [Jordan and O'Malley, 2007]. Since SERMs block a subset of estrogen effects, they may be more desirable drugs than GnRH and aromatase inhibitors due to their greater specificity and fewer side effects.

It is likely that increased knowledge of the molecular mechanisms of the post-transcriptional effects of estrogen will be another step towards therapeutic targeting of known subsets of estrogen-responsive genes. It is possible to target proteins involved in post-transcriptional regulation either by using reagents like short interfering RNAs to down-regulate the protein and reverse its effects on mRNA stability. For the proteins that regulate mRNA stability by binding directly to cis-elements on the mRNA, oligonucleotide mimics of the cis-element (also called "RNA decoys") could be used to bind and sequester those RNA-binding proteins and interrupt the proteins' effect on mRNA lifespan and function [Makeyev et al., 2002]. For example, if uteri were treated with the ER mRNA regions responsible for its stabilization (such as MEMSS), the AUF1p45 and other binding proteins could be sequestered and unable to stabilize ER mRNA. This would block the up-regulation of the expression of the ER gene, as well as the genes it subsequently up-regulates. This approach is unique because it could spare basal influences of estrogens so that bone, brain and circulatory system health would be maintained.

The elucidation of the molecular mechanisms by which microRNAs regulate the stability and/or translation of target mRNAs opens even more new therapeutic avenues for altering both normal and abnormal physiology of animal tissues. Recent advances in oligonucleotide therapeutics and gene therapy approaches make it feasible to either up- or down-regulate key microRNAs in cell culture and, subsequently, in vivo [Esau and Monia, 2007; Ford and Cheng, 2008; Zhao et al., 2008]. One group called its antisense microRNAs "antagomirs" and used them successfully in mice to down-regulate an individual microRNA [Krutzfeldt et al., 2005]. A particular microRNA might be targeted by an antisense RNA to reverse the actions of the microRNA on expression of critical genes. In another example, down-regulation of miR-221 and -222 by antisense RNAs increased ER levels in breast cancer cells [Zhao et al., 2008]. This restored estrogen-dependent cell growth as well as sensitivity to growth inhibition by the SERM tamoxifen. This may be a useful approach to treat tamoxifen-resistant breast cancer in women. Alternatively, therapies might increase concentration of microRNAs that act as tumor suppressors, like miR-17-5p in breast cancer [Hossain et al., 2006]. As our knowledge of the post-transcriptional effects of estrogens on individual genes and sets of gene products grows, so will our ability to control physiology through them in order to enhance human and animal health.

CONCLUSION

As discussed above, the many post-transcriptional actions of estrogens are an important component of their effects on the expression of specific genes. Some of these estrogen actions appear to be central to aspects of normal physiology, as well as to the development and progression of estrogen-dependent diseases including uterine and breast cancers. These effects may occur by estrogen-induced increases in the transcription of genes encoding RNAbinding proteins and/or microRNAs. Estrogens could also activate RNA-binding proteins, such as AUF1p45, by post-translational mechanisms such as dephosphorylation [Proia et al., 2006]. As we elucidate the molecular mechanisms by which estrogens regulate gene expression post-transcriptionally, we will reveal new targets and approaches for therapeutic interventions in estrogen-dependent physiology.

REFERENCES

Adams, B.D., Furneaux, H., White, B.A., 2007. The micro-ribonucleic acid (miRNA) miR-206 targets the human estrogen receptor-alpha (ERalpha) and represses ERalpha messenger RNA and protein expression in breast cancer cell lines. *Mol. Endocrinol.* 21, 1132-1147.

Arao, Y., Kikuchi, A., Ikeda, K., Nomoto, S., Horiguchi, H., Kayama, F., 2002. A+U-rich-element RNA-binding factor 1/heterogeneous nuclear ribonucleoprotein D gene expression is regulated by oestrogen in the rat uterus. *Biochemical. Journal.* 361, 125-132.

Arao, Y., Kikuchi, A., Kishida, M., Yonekura, M., Inoue, A., Yasuda, S., Wada, S., Ikeda, K., Kayama, F., 2004. Stability of A+U-rich element binding factor 1 (AUF1)-binding messenger ribonucleic acid correlates with the subcellular relocalization of AUF1 in the rat uterus upon estrogen treatment. *Mol. Endocrinol* 18, 2255-2267.

Arnold, S.F., Melamed, M., Vorojeikina, D.P., Notides, A.C., Sasson, S., 1997. Estradiol-binding mechanism and binding capacity of the human estrogen receptor is regulated by tyrosine phosphorylation. *Mol. Endocrinol.* 11, 48-53.

Baek, D., Villen, J., Shin, C., Camargo, F.D., Gygi, S.P., Bartel, D.P., 2008. The impact of microRNAs on protein output.[see comment]. *Nature* 455, 64-71.

Bhattacharyya, S.N., Habermacher, R., Martine, U., Closs, E.I., Filipowicz, W., 2006. Relief of microRNA-mediated translational repression in human cells subjected to stress. *Cell* 125, 1111-1124.

Boren, T., Xiong, Y., Hakam, A., Wenham, R., Apte, S., Wei, Z., Kamath, S., Chen, D.T., Dressman, H., Lancaster, J.M., 2008. MicroRNAs and their target messenger RNAs associated with endometrial carcinogenesis. *Gynecol. Oncol.* 110, 206-215.

Chakrabarty, A., Tranguch, S., Daikoku, T., Jensen, K., Furneaux, H., Dey, S.K., 2007. MicroRNA regulation of cyclooxygenase-2 during embryo implantation. *Proc. Natl.Acad. Sci. USA* 104, 15144-15149.

Cheadle, C., Fan, J., Cho-Chung, Y.S., Werner, T., Ray, J., Do, L., Gorospe, M., Becker, K.G., 2005. Control of gene expression during T cell activation: alternate regulation of mRNA transcription and mRNA stability. *BMC Genomics* 6, 75.

Chen, C.Y., Shyu, A.B., 1995. AU-rich elements: characterization and importance in mRNA degradation. *Trends Biochem. Sci.* 20, 465-470.

Chen, C.Y., Xu, N., Shyu, A.B., 2002. Highly selective actions of HuR in antagonizing AU-rich element-mediated mRNA destabilization. *Mol. Cell Biol.* 22, 7268-7278.

Chu, I., Arnaout, A., Loiseau, S., Sun, J., Seth, A., McMahon, C., Chun, K., Hennessy, B., Mills, G.B., Nawaz, Z., Slingerland, J.M., 2007. Src promotes estrogen-dependent estrogen receptor alpha proteolysis in human breast cancer. *J. Clin. Invest* 117, 2205-2215.

Ciesla, J., 2006. Metabolic enzymes that bind RNA: yet another level of cellular regulatory network? *Acta Biochim. Pol.* 53, 11-32.

Cohen, A., Shmoish, M., Levi, L., Cheruti, U., Levavi-Sivan, B., Lubzens, E., 2008. Alterations in micro-ribonucleic acid expression profiles reveal a novel pathway for estrogen regulation. *Endocrinology* 149, 1687-1696.

Cramer, S.F., Patel, A., 1990. The frequency of uterine leiomyomas. *Am. J. Clin. Pathol.* 94, 435-438.

Cunningham, K.S., Dodson, R.E., Nagel, M.A., Shapiro, D.J., Schoenberg, D.R., 2000. Vigilin binding selectively inhibits cleavage of the vitellogenin mRNA 3'-untranslated region by the mRNA endonuclease polysomal ribonuclease 1. *Proc. Natl. Acad. Sci. USA* 97, 12498-12502.

Cunningham, K.S., Hanson, M.N., Schoenberg, D.R., 2001. Polysomal ribonuclease 1 exists in a latent form on polysomes prior to estrogen activation of mRNA decay. *Nucleic Acids* Research 29, 1156-1162.

Dodson, R.E., Shapiro, D.J., 2002. Regulation of pathways of mRNA destabilization and stabilization. *Progress in Nucleic Acid Research and Molecular Biology* 72, 129-164.

el Meskini, R., Delfino, C., Boudouresque, F., Hery, M., Oliver, C., Ouafik, L., 1997. Estrogen regulation of peptidylglycine alpha-amidating monooxygenase expression in anterior pituitary gland. *Endocrinology* 138, 379-388.

Esau, C.C., Monia, B.P., 2007. Therapeutic potential for microRNAs. *Adv. Drug Deliv. Rev.* 59, 101-114.

Farnell, Y.Z., Ing, N.H., 2003a. The effects of estradiol and selective estrogen receptor modulators on gene expression and messenger RNA stability in immortalized sheep endometrial stromal cells and human endometrial adenocarcinoma cells. *Journal ofSteroid Biochemistry and Molecular Biology* 84, 453-461.

Farnell, Y.Z., Ing, N.H., 2003b. Endometrial effects of selective estrogen receptor modulators (SERMs) on estradiol-responsive gene expression are gene and cell-specific. *Journal ofSteroid Biochemistry and Molecular Biology* 84, 513-526.

Farnell, Y.Z., Ing, N.H., 2003c. Myometrial effects of selective estrogen receptor modulators on estradiol-responsive gene expression are gene and cell-specific. *Journal of SteroidBiochemistry and Molecular Biology* 84, 527-536.

Foekens, J.A., Sieuwerts, A.M., Smid, M., Look, M.P., de Weerd, V., Boersma, A.W., Klijn, J.G., Wiemer, E.A., Martens, J.W., 2008. Four miRNAs associated with aggressiveness of lymph node-negative, estrogen receptor-positive human breast cancer. *Proc. Natl.Acad. Sci. USA* 105, 13021-13026.

Ford, L.P., Cheng, A., 2008. Using synthetic precursor and inhibitor miRNAs to understand miRNA function. *Methods Mol. Biol.* 419, 289-301.

Friend, K.E., Resnick, E.M., Ang, L.W., Shupnik, M.A., 1997. Specific modulation of estrogen receptor mRNA isoforms in rat pituitary throughout the estrous cycle and in response to steroid hormones. *Mol. Cell Endocrinol.* 131, 147-155.

Grimson, A., Farh, K.K., Johnston, W.K., Garrett-Engele, P., Lim, L.P., Bartel, D.P., 2007. MicroRNA targeting specificity in mammals: determinants beyond seed pairing. *Mol.Cell* 27, 91-105.

Gurates, B., Bulun, S.E., 2003. Endometriosis: the ultimate hormonal disease. *Semin. ReprodMed.* 21, 125-134.

Hammond, S.M., 2006. RNAi, microRNAs, and human disease. *Cancer ChemotherPharmacol.* 58 Suppl 1, s63-68.

Hossain, A., Kuo, M.T., Saunders, G.F., 2006. Mir-17-5p regulates breast cancer cell proliferation by inhibiting translation of AIB1 mRNA. Mol. *Cell Biol.* 26, 8191-8201.

Ikeda, S., Nakamura, K., Kogure, K., Omori, Y., Yamashita, S., Kubota, K., Mizutani, T., Miyamoto, K., Minegishi, T., 2008. Effect of estrogen on the expression of luteinizing hormone-human chorionic gonadotropin receptor messenger ribonucleic acid in cultured rat granulosa cells. *Endocrinology* 149, 1524-1533.

Ing, N.H., 2005a. Steroid hormones regulate gene expression post-transcriptionally by altering the stabilities of messenger RNAs. *Biol. Reprod* 72, 1290-1296.

Ing, N.H., 2005b. Steroid hormones regulate gene expression posttranscriptionally by altering the stabilities of messenger RNAs. *Biol. Reprod.* 72, 1290-1296.

Ing, N.H., Massuto, D.A., Jaeger, L.A., 2008. Estradiol up-regulates AUF1p45 binding to stabilizing regions within the 3'-untranslated region of estrogen receptor alpha mRNA. *J. Biol. Chem.* 283, 1764-1772.

Ing, N.H., Ott, T.L., 1999. Estradiol up-regulates estrogen receptor-alpha messenger ribonucleic acid in sheep endometrium by increasing its stability. *Biol. Reprod* 60, 134-139.

Ing, N.H., Robertson J. A., 1999. *Regulation of hormone receptor gene expression.* Springer-Verlag, New York.

Iorio, M.V., Ferracin, M., Liu, C.G., Veronese, A., Spizzo, R., Sabbioni, S., Magri, E., Pedriali, M., Fabbri, M., Campiglio, M., Menard, S., Palazzo, J.P., Rosenberg, A., Musiani, P., Volinia, S., Nenci, I., Calin, G.A., Querzoli, P., Negrini, M., Croce, C.M., 2005. MicroRNA gene expression deregulation in human breast cancer. *Cancer Res.* 65, 7065-7070.

Ioshikhes, I., Roy, S., Sen, C.K., 2007. Algorithms for mapping of mRNA targets for microRNA. *DNA Cell Biol.* 26, 265-272.

Jackson, R.J., Standart, N., 2007. How do microRNAs regulate gene expression? *Sci. STKE* 2007, re1.

Jay, C., Nemunaitis, J., Chen, P., Fulgham, P., Tong, A.W., 2007. miRNA profiling for diagnosis and prognosis of human cancer. *DNA Cell Biol.* 26, 293-300.

Jiang, Q., Wang, Y., Hao, Y., Juan, L., Teng, M., Zhang, X., Li, M., Wang, G., Liu, Y., 2009. miR2Disease: a manually curated database for microRNA deregulation in human disease. *Nucleic Acids Res.* 37, D98-D104.

Jing, Q., Huang, S., Guth, S., Zarubin, T., Motoyama, A., Chen, J., Di Padova, F., Lin, S.C., Gram, H., Han, J., 2005. Involvement of microRNA in AU-rich element-mediated mRNA instability. *Cell* 120, 623-634.

Jordan, V.C., O'Malley, B.W., 2007. Selective estrogen-receptor modulators and antihormonal resistance in breast cancer. *J. Clin. Oncol.* 25, 5815-5824.

Kedde, M., Strasser, M.J., Boldajipour, B., Oude Vrielink, J.A., Slanchev, K., le Sage, C., Nagel, R., Voorhoeve, P.M., van Duijse, J., Orom, U.A., Lund, A.H., Perrakis, A., Raz, E., Agami, R., 2007. RNA-binding protein Dnd1 inhibits microRNA access to target mRNA.[see comment]. *Cell* 131, 1273-1286.

Keene, J.D., 2007. RNA regulons: coordination of post-transcriptional events. *Nat. Rev.Genet.* 8, 533-543.

Kenealy, M.R., Flouriot, G., Sonntag-Buck, V., Dandekar, T., Brand, H., Gannon, F., 2000. The 3'-untranslated region of the human estrogen receptor alpha gene mediates rapid messenger ribonucleic acid turnover. *Endocrinology* 141, 2805-2813.

Ketting, R.F., 2007. A dead end for microRNAs. [comment]. *Cell* 131, 1226-1227.

Kim, S., Lee, U.J., Kim, M.N., Lee, E.J., Kim, J.Y., Lee, M.Y., Choung, S., Kim, Y.J., Choi, Y.C., 2008. MicroRNA miR-199a* regulates the MET proto-oncogene and the downstream extracellular signal-regulated kinase 2 (ERK2). *J. Biol. Chem.* 283, 18158-18166.

Kimura, N., Arai, K., Sahara, Y., Suzuki, H., 1994. Estradiol transcriptionally and posttranscriptionally up-regulates thyrotropin-releasing hormone receptor messenger ribonucleic acid in rat pituitary cells. *Endocrinology* 134, 432-440.

Kovalchuk, O., Tryndyak, V.P., Montgomery, B., Boyko, A., Kutanzi, K., Zemp, F., Warbritton, A.R., Latendresse, J.R., Kovalchuk, I., Beland, F.A., Pogribny, I.P., 2007. Estrogen-induced rat breast carcinogenesis is characterized by alterations in DNA methylation, histone modifications and aberrant microRNA expression. *Cell Cycle* 6, 2010-2018.

Krutzfeldt, J., Rajewsky, N., Braich, R., Rajeev, K.G., Tuschl, T., Manoharan, M., Stoffel, M., 2005. Silencing of microRNAs in vivo with 'antagomirs'. *Nature* 438, 685-689.

Kyrpides, N.C., Ouzounis, C.A., 1995. Nucleic acid-binding metabolic enzymes: living fossils of stereochemical interactions? *J. Mol. Evol.* 40, 564-569.

Landgraf, P., Rusu, M., Sheridan, R., Sewer, A., Iovino, N., Aravin, A., Pfeffer, S., Rice, A., Kamphorst, A.O., Landthaler, M., Lin, C., Socci, N.D., Hermida, L., Fulci, V., Chiaretti, S., Foa, R., Schliwka, J., Fuchs, U., Novosel, A., Muller, R.U., Schermer, B., Bissels, U., Inman, J., Phan, Q., Chien, M., Weir, D.B., Choksi, R., De Vita, G., Frezzetti, D., Trompeter, H.I., Hornung, V., Teng, G., Hartmann, G., Palkovits, M., Di Lauro, R., Wernet, P., Macino, G., Rogler, C.E., Nagle, J.W., Ju, J., Papavasiliou, F.N., Benzing, T., Lichter, P., Tam, W., Brownstein, M.J., Bosio, A., Borkhardt, A., Russo, J.J., Sander, C., Zavolan, M., Tuschl, T., 2007. A mammalian microRNA expression atlas based on small RNA library sequencing.[see comment]. *Cell* 129, 1401-1414.

Lasa, M., Mahtani, K.R., Finch, A., Brewer, G., Saklatvala, J., Clark, A.R., 2000. Regulation of cyclooxygenase 2 mRNA stability by the mitogen-activated protein kinase p38 signaling cascade. *Mol. Cell Biol.* 20, 4265-4274.

Liang, Y., Ridzon, D., Wong, L., Chen, C., 2007. Characterization of microRNA expression profiles in normal human tissues. *BMC Genomics* 8, 166.

Lodish, H.F., Zhou, B., Liu, G., Chen, C.Z., 2008. Micromanagement of the immune system by microRNAs.[erratum appears in Nat Rev Immunol. 2008 Mar;8(3):238]. *Nature RevImmunol.* 8, 120-130.

Loflin, P., Chen, C.Y., Shyu, A.B., 1999. Unraveling a cytoplasmic role for hnRNP D in the in vivo mRNA destabilization directed by the AU-rich element. *Genes and Development* 13, 1884-1897.

Lu, J., Getz, G., Miska, E.A., Alvarez-Saavedra, E., Lamb, J., Peck, D., Sweet-Cordero, A., Ebert, B.L., Mak, R.H., Ferrando, A.A., Downing, J.R., Jacks, T., Horvitz, H.R., Golub, T.R., 2005. MicroRNA expression profiles classify human cancers.[see comment]. *Nature* 435, 834-838.

Lui, W.O., Pourmand, N., Patterson, B.K., Fire, A., 2007. Patterns of known and novel small RNAs in human cervical cancer. *Cancer Res.* 67, 6031-6043.

Makeyev, A.V., Eastmond, D.L., Liebhaber, S.A., 2002. Targeting a KH-domain protein with RNA decoys. *RNA* 8, 1160-1173.

Marsh, E.E., Lin, Z., Yin, P., Milad, M., Chakravarti, D., Bulun, S.E., 2008. Differential expression of microRNA species in human uterine leiomyoma versus normal myometrium. *Fertil Steril* 89, 1771-1776.

Mathonnet, G., Fabian, M.R., Svitkin, Y.V., Parsyan, A., Huck, L., Murata, T., Biffo, S., Merrick, W.C., Darzynkiewicz, E., Pillai, R.S., Filipowicz, W., Duchaine, T.F., Sonenberg, N., 2007. MicroRNA inhibition of translation initiation in vitro by targeting the cap-binding complex eIF4F. *Science* 317, 1764-1767.

Mattie, M.D., Benz, C.C., Bowers, J., Sensinger, K., Wong, L., Scott, G.K., Fedele, V., Ginzinger, D., Getts, R., Haqq, C., 2006. Optimized high-throughput microRNA expression profiling provides novel biomarker assessment of clinical prostate and breast cancer biopsies. *Mol. Cancer* 5, 24.

Maziere, P., Enright, A.J., 2007. Prediction of microRNA targets. *Drug Discov. Today* 12, 452-458.

McKean-Cowdin, R., Feigelson, H.S., Pike, M.C., Coetzee, G.A., Kolonel, L.N., Henderson, B.E., 2001. Risk of endometrial cancer and estrogen replacement therapy history by CYP17 genotype. *Cancer Res.* 61, 848-849.

Miller, B.G., Wild, J., Stone, G.M., 1979. Effects of progesterone on the oestrogen-stimulated uterus: a comparative study of the mouse, guinea pig, rabbit and sheep. *Aust. J. Biol. Sci.* 32, 549-560.

Mitchell, D.C., Ing, N.H., 2003. Estradiol stabilizes estrogen receptor messenger ribonucleic acid in sheep endometrium via discrete sequence elements in its 3'-untranslated region. *Mol. Endocrinol.* 17, 562-574.

Moore, N.W., Miller, B.G., Trappl, M.N., 1983. Transport and development of embryos transferred to the oviducts and uteri of entire and ovariectomized ewes. *J. Reprod. Fertil* 68, 129-135.

Mukherjee, D., Gao, M., O'Connor, J.P., Raijmakers, R., Pruijn, G., Lutz, C.S., Wilusz, J., 2002. The mammalian exosome mediates the efficient degradation of mRNAs that contain AU-rich elements. *EMBO Journal* 21, 165-174.

Nagy, E., Maquat, L.E., 1998. A rule for termination-codon position within intron-containing genes: when nonsense affects RNA abundance. *Trends Biochem. Sci.* 23, 198-199.

Nair, A.K., Young, M.A., Menon, K.M., 2008. Regulation of luteinizing hormone receptor mRNA expression by mevalonate kinase--role of the catalytic center in mRNA recognition. *FEBS J.* 275, 3397-3407.

Nowak, R.A., 2001. Identification of new therapies for leiomyomas: what in vitro studies can tell us. *Clin. Obstet. Gynecol.* 44, 327-334.

Palmiter, R.D., 1972. Regulation of protein synthesis in chick oviduct. II. Modulation of polypeptide elongation and initiation rates by estrogen and progesterone. *J. Biol. Chem.* 247, 6770-6780.

Pan, Q., Luo, X., Toloubeydokhti, T., Chegini, N., 2007. The expression profile of micro-RNA in endometrium and endometriosis and the influence of ovarian steroids on their expression. *Mol. Hum. Reprod.* 13, 797-806.

Parker, R., Song, H., 2004. The enzymes and control of eukaryotic mRNA turnover. *Nature Structural and Molecular Biology* 11, 121-127.

Proia, D.A., Nannenga, B.W., Donehower, L.A., Weigel, N.L., 2006. Dual roles for the phosphatase PPM1D in regulating progesterone receptor function. *J. Biol. Chem.* 281, 7089-7101.

Robertson, J.A., Zhang, Y., Ing, N.H., 2001. ICI 182,780 acts as a partial agonist and antagonist of estradiol effects in specific cells of the sheep uterus. *Journal of SteroidBiochemistry and Molecular Biology* 77, 281-287.

Rodriguez-Pinon, M., Meikle, A., Tasende, C., Sahlin, L., Garofalo, E.G., 2005. Differential estradiol effects on estrogen and progesterone receptors expression in the oviduct and cervix of immature ewes. *Domestic Animal Endocrinology* 28, 442-450.

Saceda, M., Lindsey, R.K., Solomon, H., Angeloni, S.V., Martin, M.B., 1998. Estradiol regulates estrogen receptor mRNA stability. *Journal of Steroid Biochemistry andMolecular Biology* 66, 113-120.

Saxena, S., Jonsson, Z.O., Dutta, A., 2003. Small RNAs with imperfect match to endogenous mRNA repress translation. Implications for off-target activity of small inhibitory RNA in mammalian cells. *J. Biol. Chem.* 278, 44312-44319.

Seaver, S.S., 1981. The effects of sequential hormone treatment on ovalbumin synthesis in chick oviduct: a possible example of translation regulation. *J. Steroid Biochem.* 14, 949-957.

Sela-Brown, A., Silver, J., Brewer, G., Naveh-Many, T., 2000. Identification of AUF1 as a parathyroid hormone mRNA 3'-untranslated region-binding protein that determines parathyroid hormone mRNA stability. *J. Biol. Chem.* 275, 7424-7429.

Sengupta, S., Jang, B.C., Wu, M.T., Paik, J.H., Furneaux, H., Hla, T., 2003. The RNA-binding protein HuR regulates the expression of cyclooxygenase-2. *J. Biol. Chem.* 278, 25227-25233.

Sun, M., Estrov, Z., Ji, Y., Coombes, K.R., Harris, D.H., Kurzrock, R., 2008. Curcumin (diferuloylmethane) alters the expression profiles of microRNAs in human pancreatic cancer cells. *Mol. Cancer Ther* 7, 464-473.

Tsai, M.J., Clark, J.H., Schrader, W.T., O'Malley, B.W., 1998. Mechanisms of action of hormones that act as transcription factors. Saunders, Philadelphia.

Vasudevan, N., Pfaff, D.W., 2008. Non-genomic actions of estrogens and their interaction with genomic actions in the brain. *Front Neuroendocrinol* 29, 238-257.

Wagner, B.J., DeMaria, C.T., Sun, Y., Wilson, G.M., Brewer, G., 1998. Structure and genomic organization of the human AUF1 gene: alternative pre-mRNA splicing generates four protein isoforms. *Genomics* 48, 195-202.

Wang, L., Nair, A.K., Menon, K.M., 2007a. Ribonucleic acid binding protein-mediated regulation of luteinizing hormone receptor expression in granulosa cells: relationship to sterol metabolism. *Mol. Endocrinol.* 21, 2233-2241.

Wang, T., Zhang, X., Obijuru, L., Laser, J., Aris, V., Lee, P., Mittal, K., Soteropoulos, P., Wei, J.J., 2007b. A micro-RNA signature associated with race, tumor size, and target gene activity in human uterine leiomyomas. *Genes Chromosomes Cancer* 46, 336-347.

Watson, C.S., Alyea, R.A., Jeng, Y.J., Kochukov, M.Y., 2007. Nongenomic actions of low concentration estrogens and xenoestrogens on multiple tissues. *Mol. Cell Endocrinol.* 274, 1-7.

Whelly, S.M., Barker, K.L., 1974. Early effect of estradiol on the peptide elongation rate by uterine ribosomes. *Biochemistry* 13, 341-346.

Wilson, G.M., Sutphen, K., Bolikal, S., Chuang, K.Y., Brewer, G., 2001. Thermodynamics and kinetics of Hsp70 association with A + U-rich mRNA-destabilizing sequences. *J.Biol. Chem.* 276, 44450-44456.

Wu, L., Belasco, J.G., 2008. Let me count the ways: mechanisms of gene regulation by miRNAs and siRNAs. *Mol. Cell* 29, 1-7.

Xu, N., Chen, C.Y., Shyu, A.B., 2001. Versatile role for hnRNP D isoforms in the differential regulation of cytoplasmic mRNA turnover. *Mol. Cell Biol.* 21, 6960-6971.

Yan, L.X., Huang, X.F., Shao, Q., Huang, M.Y., Deng, L., Wu, Q.L., Zeng, Y.X., Shao, J.Y., 2008. MicroRNA miR-21 overexpression in human breast cancer is associated with advanced clinical stage, lymph node metastasis and patient poor prognosis. *RNA* 14, 2348-2360.

Zhao, J.J., Lin, J., Yang, H., Kong, W., He, L., Ma, X., Coppola, D., Cheng, J.Q., 2008. MicroRNA-221/222 negatively regulates estrogen receptor alpha and is associated with tamoxifen resistance in breast cancer. *J. Biol. Chem.* 283, 31079-31086.

Zhao, Z., Chang, F.C., Furneaux, H.M., 2000. The identification of an endonuclease that cleaves within an HuR binding site in mRNA. *Nucleic. Acids Research* 28, 2695-2701.

D

G

H

I

R